CW01080397

A Study Guide
to
Nursing Theories

A supplement to
A Study Guide to Nursing Theories

**GERT
HUNINK**

The
Vijverberg
Evaluation Instrument
for Nursing Theories

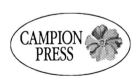

Campion Press
384 Lanark Road
Edinburgh EH13 0LX

A Description

A1 How does the theoretician describe his own background and approach, and how is she or he described by other authors? Consider topics such as training and experience (including work-experience) and other factors.

A2 With what aim or purpose in mind was the theory formulated?

A3 Has the theory developed through time, or is it (at the moment) a one-off presentation? If the theory has developed outline the course it has taken, including dates if possible.

A4 Is there a relationship between this theory and other theories or ideas? To what extent is it based on the knowledge of other authors' work or theories?

A5 On what ideological or philosophical principles and assumptions is the theory explicitly based? What is the nature of these principles and assumptions?

A6 What are the theoretician's ideas about scientific nursing theories, about the process of theory development and about the application and testing of theories in general? In what ways does she or he want to contribute to this?

B Analysis and criticism

B1 In what ways have the theorist's experiences, training and background had a positive or negative effect on the theory?

B2 Describe how you feel about the reasons and the aims behind the theory. Does it seem to you that these aims will be met?

B3 How would you assess the theory's development? Is this development an improvement? If there has been no development so far, in what ways do you think it would be useful or even necessary?

B4 To what extent is the theory based on other theories? Does it use the ideas of other authors without acknowledging them?

B5 On what principles or assumptions is the theory implicitly based? What consequences could the principles or assumptions, both implicit and explicit, have? What are their advantages and disadvantages?

B6 How does the theorist's view agree with or differ from that of other theorists? What are the consequences of this view? Is the theory itself in agreement with the theorist's view? Is it, in its present form, suitable for the aim the theorist has in mind or would a different kind of theory be more suitable?

A7 What type of theory is it with regard to
- the function of the theory,
- the level of the theory, and
- the range of the theory?

B7 Is the theory at a suitable level for its aim? Would it be possible to develop it further, to a higher level? Would it be possible to link the theory to others with a different range? Explain how.

A8 What does the theory say about the following central concepts ('meta-paradigms') and how they interrelate?
a: the human being, person and patient
b: health/illness
c: environment
d: nursing

B8 In what ways do the descriptions of the four central concepts agree with the views of other theorists and how do they differ, both according to the theorist himself and to other authors? Has the relationship between them been clearly and logically described? What are the consequences of defining the concepts in this particular way?

A9 What important concepts is the theory specifically based on? What concrete examples are given?

B9 What are the most important characteristics of the concepts? Have the concepts themselves been clearly defined? How are they distinguished from related or synonymous concepts? Is this description recognizable in the practical situation? Is it used consistently?

A10 How do the most important propositions or statements relate these concepts to each other?

B10 What is the nature of the relationship between the concepts? Are the statements or propositions logical? Have they been well enough argued? Is it possible to test them? To what extent are they based on empirical data?

A11 Is the Nursing Process described? If so, what is said about it? If not, what other guidelines are given about the practical situation? Are there any other specific guides given about the theory's usage?

B11 What differences and similarities are there between this and the work of other authors with respect to the formulation, content and practice of the Nursing Process? Can it be applied directly within the practical nursing situation?

A12 What does the theory say about its generality; or where and when it can be used? Does it distinguish between the different fields of nursing, or is it thought to be equally useful in all the different fields?

A13 What is known about how the theory (or parts of it) can be applied within the different fields and the levels at which it can be applied (administration, care or research)?

A14 Does the theory say anything about the following?
a: Nursing in general
b: Nursing education
c: Nursing administration
d: Nursing research.

A15 What criticism or support has the theory received? Who has offered this commentary, and what were the arguments and motives used?

B12 To which fields or areas of care does the theory principally appear to be applicable? Can it also be used in situations other than those indicated?

B13 What would be your evaluation of the application of this theory? Does the way in which it can be used agree with the intentions of the theory and those of the theoretician her or himself?

B14 To what extent and in what way are nursing, and nursing training, management and research. discussed? What consequences might this have? How does it compare with the work of other theoreticians? Is the theory based on general values as they are formulated in, for instance, the professional codes?

B15 Is the positive or negative criticism of the various parts of the theory unambiguous? Is this criticism related to essential or less essential parts of the theory, or to the theory as a whole? How would you analyse and evaluate the criticism? What are your reasons and arguments for this analysis?

Conclusion
What general conclusions can you make by way of summary? What are the strengths and weaknesses of the theory? Give your own opinion.

A Study Guide to Nursing Theories

Gert Hunink

Campion Press, Edinburgh

1995

British Library Cataloguing in Publication Data:

Hunink, G.
    Study Guide to Nursing Theories
    I. Title
    610.7301

ISBN 1 873732 15 5

This publication was initally produced with the co-operation of the
Department of Contract Activities of the Vijverberg-Felua College for
Higher Education in Ede, The Netherlands

© 1995 Campion Press

Published by Campion Press
384 Lanark Road, Edinburgh EH13 0LX

Designed and typeset in 10/12pt Palatino by Artisan Graphics, Edinburgh
Printed and bound by Bell and Bain, Glasgow.

Preface

This book aims to be an *introduction* to nursing theorizing and an *aid* to the
practical application of the theories produced. It was preceded by two
reports, which had their foundations in a study group at the Vijverberg-
Felua College in Ede, The Netherlands. The aim of this group, which
consisted of a psychologist, a philosopher and a nursing scientist, was to
clarify the process of theory development in nursing, and to make
theories easier to handle for both tutors and students within nursing
training at this college.

To achieve this, the study group first of all attempted to clarify the
terminology in use with respect to theories (often, there is vagueness or
disagreement about the definition and application of some of the central
concepts). Then the group considered the different aspects which can be
distinguished in theories, and this helped to map some points of decision
related, for instance, to the views the theories are based on, and others
concerned with how and when a theory can be applied. On this basis,
points of evaluation were formulated. Taken together these points consti-
tuted an 'evaluation instrument' which can be used to assess a theory.

Several evaluation instruments are already in use in publications concerned with nursing science (see also the appendices). The study group
had no intention of re-inventing the wheel: the existing instruments have
been used in the search for points of evaluation that can be used within
nursing training in a college of higher education.

The group did not claim to be either complete or scientific in its achieve-
ments; neither does this book make such a claim. The first report
appeared in January 1993, and a revised version was published a year
later. The reports and the 'Vijverberg Evaluation Instrument for Nursing
Theories' (the Vijverberg ENT) have proved effective in the college where
they were devised.

This book and the evaluation instrument can be used by individuals or
small groups of tutors and/or students as part of the training process. It

may also prove useful outside the training college, in for example nursing practice or nursing administration. Within an organisation it can enable an individual, a study group or a team to use nursing theories effectively within the specific work situation.

We hope to make a constructive contribution to developments in this field, and to promote the fruitful application of theories. For this reason, the reader is encouraged to read and use this book critically and think with us about the inspiring profession of nursing. Rather than learning and reproducing the contents of this book, we would like the reader to accept the *challenge* of thinking creatively about her own profession, or future profession. As a result, she will find that much of what appears to be straightforward and obvious turns out not to be straightforward at all! The nursing profession changes continually, and you can contribute to its change.

By now, changes and additions have been made to the original text of the first edition. Nursing is a growing profession, and so is the development of theories. It is likely that a revised edition will appear in due course, and I would welcome comments and suggestions!

I would like to conclude this preface with a few words of gratitude. In particular, I would like to thank my colleagues Wil Doornenbal and Peter Blokhuis, who were involved in the first report which was mainly geared towards our own nursing training course. I would also like to thank Bart Cusveller for his critical comments on both the first report and this book. There are, of course, many other people I would like to mention here, but I will restrict myself to thanking, as a group, the staff members of the Nursing Science Faculty in Maastricht for the stimulating course which prompted me to deeper thought about my profession, and my colleagues and students on the nursing training course in Ede and the Nursing Science course in Utrecht. I hope that many more inspiring discussions will follow. Finally, I would like to thank Rita and our children, and warn them that this book is not intended to be the last word on the subject!

Gert Hunink

Amersfoort, 1994

Contents

Contents

Introduction

We can no longer deny that, in nursing, scientific research and theories are increasingly becoming important aspects of the profession. This book concentrates on nursing theory development (process) and theories (product), and tries to answer some of the questions surrounding theories, what they are, what their uses are and what we can do with them[1].

Florence Nightingale's ideas are generally considered to be the beginnings of modern nursing. Her *Notes on Nursing* (1859) was like a lone tree in a desert. However, the production of nursing theories has boomed since the 1950s, particularly in the United States. One of the aims of theories is to give direction in the practical situation, but when different theories point in different directions they can make things more complex rather than more straightforward. Many nurses, in any case, find it difficult to get used to the increasingly scientific nature of nursing. They find it hard to see the wood for the trees.

But what use can we actually make of these theories? Their practical application in nursing is still in its infancy, due partly to the somewhat abstract character of theories and partly to unfamiliarity within the nursing profession. It also appears that nurses are more inclined to act than to think about their profession.

The 'wood of theories' will soon seem like an impenetrable *jungle*. In it, though, can be found much that is worth the effort of the search. This book aims to be a *guide* through this jungle. First, we will discuss the relationship between nursing and science, the importance of theories and the usefulness of evaluation.

---

1 We will not, in this work, elaborate on the various definitions of and distinctions between concepts like *theory, model* and *view*. We will use the word 'theory' in a broad sense, in which different definitions of the concept will be contained (this is discussed further in section 2.1 and Appendix 3). Appendix 3 also discusses some other terms used within nursing science, and should be consulted for a brief explanation of these terms.

We will then discuss how various theoretical aspects of theories can be evaluated, and present an 'evaluation instrument' based on our findings (see Appendix 1). This instrument is an *aid* to the analysis and comparison of various theories, and will allow us to expand our knowledge of, and insight into, the differences and similarities between theories. We will examine more closely both their practical application in nursing practice, and their implicit and explicit assumptions, including for example the philosophical foundations on which the theory is based.

This is a particularly important task for nurses in training who, once they have come to grips with theorizing and have learned to look critically at the different theories, will be able to apply these theories in the practical situation of nursing. There can be more of a problem when the nurse is already qualified and working, and in such situations, we need to appeal to the nurse's personal interest and to schemes for extra training. However, this book should also be helpful to them, and it will also be useful to nursing managers. It is our aim that the reader, after studying the book and using the evaluation instrument, will be better equipped to think about and discuss theorizing and its use in nursing practice and to read and analyse theoretical publications.

The book discusses the development of theories in nursing and introduces the differences in types of theories. It also looks at their usefulness, their application, and how they can be evaluated. For comparison we have included two other evaluation instruments in the appendices. Appendix 3 discusses a few of the concepts concerned with theorizing, and appendix 4 lists some of the primary literature of theories. Finally, we include a few tables which either come from the relevant literature, or have been compiled by us on the basis of this literature. These tables contain useful information about the various theories and are meant as an aid for collecting further information. The book concludes with a general bibliography.

The order in which we present this material will not appeal equally to all our readers. One person will want to know first what is meant by 'theory' or 'science', another may wonder why theory development is necessary, and a third will want to know why it is necessary to evaluate and what should be evaluated. The chapters are therefore written in such a way that the reader can choose the order in which he wants to work through them.

A word of advice to the reader: do not be put off by the various new or unfamiliar words that are used. Give yourself, and the scientific literature of nursing, a chance. You will soon get used to it!

The Author

From 1980, Gert Hunink took part in in-service training in general nursing at the St Elisabeth Hospital (now Hospital Eemland) in Amersfoort, The Netherlands. After completing his training he worked in an Intensive Care/Coronary Care Department for five years. During this period he began studies at the University of Limburg in Maastricht, specialising in Nursing Science, and while a student he was appointed Nursing Researcher with a research grant from the Netherlands Heart Association for a period of two years (1989–1991). Since graduating he has worked as a tutor at the Vijverberg-Felua College in Ede, a Christian institution for higher education, teaching in both the full-time and part-time nursing training courses and providing supervision and guidance to students on work placement. He also provides support to students working on their final project. He also carries out applied research for the Department of Contract Activities, and develops and presents courses. In addition, he is involved as a tutor in the part-time Nursing Science programme at the University of Utrecht.

CHAPTER ONE

Nursing and Science

The origins of nursing science (the science that occupies itself with nursing) can be found in the United States. In this chapter we will briefly discuss the position of science within nursing and the position which nursing science holds, or aspires to, within the whole of nursing. What is the place of the development of theories? We will also point out here the limitations of science in general and the place of science within society.

1.1 The position of nursing science

Nursing science does not aim to look down from an ivory tower upon the practical situation of nursing care, administration and education. Rather, it contributes to the whole of the nursing field, the development of professionalism within nursing, and the improvement of the quality of care. The central element within the nursing field is the delivery of nursing care in practice. Neither nursing science, nor nursing administration nor education, has a reason for existence without nursing practice. Figure 1.1 shows how this can be reflected in a diagram.

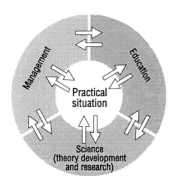

Figure 1.1 *This diagram shows how nursing practice, management, education and nursing science interrelate. We could draw another circle around the outer circle with the professional organizations, politics, and government bodies.*

Besides being concerned with university education, nursing science especially involves theory development and scientific research. Theory development and research can be regarded as the instruments of science which interact.

For example, research into patient satisfaction with the care they receive produces knowledge, and through theory development this knowledge can be placed in a 'framework'. Conversely, a theory about the needs of patients can give rise to research in the practical situation.

Nursing science can be defined as a 'practical science', and it should be regarded as an *integral part* of the nursing discipline. Its principal aim is the 'satisfactory delivery of care'. It is generally assumed that the scientific approach contributes to professionalism in nursing and to the quality of nursing care. At the core of nursing science is the need to research the action and thinking associated with nursing and to base this on scientific theories. This means that the nursing profession continually looks critically at its conduct and the reasoning behind this conduct.

It is interesting that within the profession two opposing views can be found. On the one hand, there are those who embrace nursing science as if it is the fount of all wisdom, and on the other there are those who strongly reject it. The latter group would say that the nursing profession is primarily a practical profession, concerned with 'doing'. They are not interested in 'pseudo-intellectuals who only think about the profession from behind a desk, who have forgotten what a patient looks like and who do not know how to get the work done'. A middle course seems to be the most realistic approach. Nursing science can be regarded as a necessary condition for the professionalization of nursing, but it is not the only one. However, the profession can use it to its advantage and it is therefore important to bridge the gap between 'practice' and 'theory or science'.

Much of the nurse's knowledge has traditionally been based on the combination of a few sources:

— authority
— personal experience
— trial and error
— tradition and custom
— logical reasoning
— other scientific disciplines

Knowledge from these sources is not necessarily wrong. However, they are not always equally sound. This can mean that some nursing interventions are superfluous or even harmful. Sometimes, these kinds of interventions are jokingly called 'nursing *rituals*' (Walsh and Ford, 1990). Those who require our care can expect from the nursing profession that it looks critically at what it does and why. Nursing science, in cooperation with the nursing profession, administration and the practical situation, can make an important contribution to this. Our profession and those who need us deserve this, and nursing science can help us to achieve it.

1.2 Limitations of science

We should bear in mind the restrictions of science and scientific methods. In general, a critical attitude towards science appears desirable. This means we should recognize the relative importance of 'science' as one method for collecting, organizing and applying knowledge, and gaining some insight into our complex reality. This will contribute to our thinking critically about reality and how it interacts with the research done on it.

Within science in general, there are different views on what is scientific and what is not (and, related to this, how true knowledge can be acquired). Over the years these views, which themselves are determined by all kinds of presuppositions, have constantly been altered. Even today, there is no consensus about them. This problem is the subject of epistemology, the science of science itself. One epistemological school which had a dominant influence in the United States (as opposed to Europe) for a long time was *neopositivism*, also called logical positivism or empiricism. Nursing science, which had just began to develop in the United States at this stage, was influenced by this school, both directly in the US and indirectly elsewhere (Grypdonck, 1981).

We regularly, therefore, come across the concept of forming a 'body of knowledge' or even a 'rock bottom of knowledge' within the scientific literature of nursing. The underlying thought is that through occupying ourselves with science we continually acquire knowledge about reality, and thus a solid foundation is laid which we can use to build on. This fits in with neopositivistic views of science. The phrase 'rock bottom of knowledge' is not always used in the sense of an unchangeable basis which is solid as a rock. Many authors bear in mind that views may change, and emphasize that knowledge often has a temporary character. Perhaps it would therefore be sensible to use the term 'body of knowledge' carefully.

Over the years, many objections have been made against the above epistemological school, and alternatives have been formulated. Other views, however, also have their limitations. Due to the different points of departure underlying different presuppositions, it seems unlikely that agreement will be reached. In spite of the status often given to science, it is still very much a human endeavour: views on reality are regulated by beliefs and norms. Thus, there is no clear border between what is real science and what is not (Reuling, 1986, p 123).

This is a fundamental discussion, both literally and figuratively, and we lack the space here to elaborate on it. Instead, we refer the reader to the abundance of literature in this field. Nevertheless, it is important for the development of nursing science to think thoroughly about science itself.

According to Grypdonck (1981), nursing scientists have 'mostly limited themselves to copying the views of others or undifferentiated eclecticism. In the latter case, views are combined which are based on different, incompatible principles'. Grypdonck states that original, epistemological thought is often lacking in nursing science. This applies to the situation in The Netherlands as well, though I personally feel that this attitude is changing — there appears to be ample opportunity for thorough discussions on science.

1.3 Science and society

We should constantly bear in mind that nursing science, and also therefore the development of theories, are closely linked to our society and to the other sciences. Science in general needs to be placed in a broader framework and nursing science should not, and will not, be developed in isolation. We must keep a close eye on developments within society, and within science in general which forms part of society. There is (or there was) a general tendency in society, and therefore also in science and the professions, to separate religion from science, and faith from work.

Thus, believing has become something very private: faith and science have become one another's opposites. This view of science has led to a situation where science has in many cases replaced religion in our society, with many people proclaiming their great faith in science. This position is gradually beginning to change, through the influence of discoveries in quantum physics and other factors (van den Beukel, 1991). So far discoveries in the field of quantum physics have had little effect, but in the near future they could cause a revolution in other fields of science, and may result in more room for religion and spirituality. This development may also infuence the development of theories, through promoting the idea of pluralism within theory development (see section 4.2).

In some of the more recent outlines of nursing theories, more attention appears to be paid to spiritual elements. Theories with a more general, 'neutral' character (especially those on the grand and middle-range level) may be replaced in the future by theories that have more ideological or spiritual colouring. This will no doubt have an effect on our views on nursing, disease and so on, and therefore also on nursing conduct. In a more general sense, there may be more room for important questions related to major areas such as the purpose and meaning of life (see also van der Bruggen, 1992, from p 216).

All of this has consequences for the daily practice of nursing. When diseases and problems are regarded as conditions which the patient has chosen either consciously or subconsciously, as Kuypers for instance argues, this means that the patient can only recover when he or she has been confronted with this fact (Kuypers, 1988).

It is a misconception, though, that a theory which has been formulated in a rather neutral way (such as Orem's) is not coloured by the author's philosophy or ideology. Concepts like self-actualisation and autonomy are based on ideological views as well. Therefore, it is certainly justifiable to take the ideological aspects of a theory into account in our evaluation and, if desired, when chosing a theory (see also Veling, 1991). It is of essential importance, though, that we evaluate in a thorough, systematic way and do the theorist justice.

CHAPTER TWO

Nursing
and Theories

It is generally accepted that modern nursing began with Florence Nightingale's 'Notes on Nursing: what it is and what it is not' in 1859. In the same period, initiatives were developed in different places in Europe which aimed to make nursing into a respectable profession; ideas concerning the package of knowledge associated with nursing were developed as well. It was only in the 1950s, though, that the development of theories for nursing really took off in the United States.

During this period of theory development there was also the development of 'borrowed theories': attempts were made to introduce theories from other sciences. But because the reality of nursing differs from, for example, social-pedagogic, medical or cultural-anthropological realities, the conviction grew that nursing should develop its own theories. Nevertheless, most theories can be fitted into broader lines of thought. Around 1980, the more influential theorists produced more definitive version of their theories, which were, to a larger extent than previously, supported by research and practical evidence.

2.1 Theories
Although it is not our intention to get entangled in a discussion about the concept of 'theory' itself, we will need to pay some attention to this briefly to prevent a few misconceptions.

The concept of 'theory' has different meanings:

1 *knowledge* from books, instructions and guidelines for the practical situation
2 as the *opposite* of 'practice' ('in theory' meaning 'not in practice')
3 as a *possible explanation*, guess, assumption or hypothesis
4 a way of looking at something, a vision

5 *scientific* meanings, eg:
— a theory as a 'law', a universal rule (eg the law of gravitation)
— as an explanation of a number of related facts
— empirically tested knowledge, or knowledge to be tested.

The word theory, then, is used to refer to very different things. Therefore, we always need to check its meaning and the context in which it is used.

Although there is not always a clear distinction between the definitions listed above, in this book we will concentrate on a more or less scientific meaning. We will not use the word in its meaning of 'knowledge from books' or 'instructions for the practical situation'.

In short, by 'theory' we will mean 'a set of statements about a part of reality'. For the sake of convenience, we will adhere to this general definition, which includes the concepts of 'views' and 'models'.

Whether or not a theory is 'scientific' is a separate point of discussion (see also sections 1.2 and 4.3).

2.2 Trends
In spite of the wide variety in nursing theories, a few trends can be distinguished in the theories developed since the 1950s. They show a degree of similarity in the following points:

1   a more *holistic* approach;
2   formulating a *domain* of nursing;
3   a more *patient-centred* approach;
4   the different stages of care are organized in a *Nursing Process*;
5   attention is paid to four *core elements*.

These trends in nursing theories correspond to a number of developments within the nursing profession. It is not easy to determine whether the developments in nursing, like the shift from working in a task-oriented way to working in a patient-centred way, are the products of the attention given to such matters in nursing theories or whether these theories themselves are the results of the changing practical situation — or, indeed, whether the two factors have influenced each other. Personally, I think that the last possibility, that there is a continuous interaction between theory and practice, is the more realistic one.

The different trends are described in more detail below, as they give a general picture of current nursing theories. They tend to affect one another. A change in the view of human beings, for instance, will affect how those who seek care are approached.

2.2.1 The holistic approach

Over the years, nurses became dissatisfied with the so-called medical model, which is based on a dualistic view of man. Cartesian dualism has led to an almost complete separation between treatment and care for the body on the one hand, and for the mind on the other. Under the influence of this dualistic view of man, nursing has seen the separate development of psychiatric and general nursing, which is comparable to their separate development in medicine. In hospitals it was often only the physical aspects of the care that were emphasized.

This dualism, or dichotomy, is attributed to Rene Descartes, a French philosopher who lived in the early 17th century. He regarded body and mind as two equally important, but separate elements (figure 2.1). Man was seen as 'a machine with a ghost inside'.

As stated above, this view of man is characteristic within the 'medical model'. Medicine has developed, following the model of the natural sciences, with its object being the human organism (even sometimes called 'the human machine', with the heart for example being regarded solely as a pump).

The nursing theories which have been developed over recent years advocate a more *holistic* approach. This means that in addition to physical factors, the social, psychological and spiritual aspects of the human condition should be emphasized as well. One result of this line of thought has been the emergence of generic training courses for nurses within full-time education.

A similar development, also called the 'integral approach', can be found in the new fields of health centre medicine and nursing home medicine.

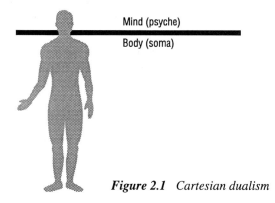

Mind (psyche)

Body (soma)

Figure 2.1 *Cartesian dualism*

'Holism' can be interpreted in different ways. Two possible interpretations are:

— *Anthropological holism*, which views the human being as a unity in itself, rather than the sum of various different parts; and

— *Cosmological holism*, which views the entire cosmos as a coherent unity. The human being is regarded as a small part of the entire universe, a 'small cog in an enormous wheel', totally influenced and determined by both the micro- and the macro-cosmos.

For the sake of completeness we should, in addition to holistic and dualistic views of mankind, also mention monistic views. A monistic view of humanity gives prominence to one particular aspect (without necessarily denying the other aspects, but by deriving them from the emphasized aspect). We can distinguish the following three principal forms (Ouweneel, 1984):

— *Materialism*, in which the psychological aspect is reducible to the physical aspect. The psychological aspect is seen as a function of the physical aspect. The entire world consists of matter only.
— *Idealism*, in which the material aspect is subordinate to the psychological aspect; it mirrors the idealistic, psychological aspect. Reality only exists in the realm of thought.
— *Neutral monism*, in which man is neither physical nor psychological, but consists of an unknown 'neutral' substance which manifests itself in different ways.

Over the centuries, mankind has philosophized about the ways in which body and mind interrelate, and many different views have been formulated. It is not always possible to make an exact distinction between monistic, dualistic and holistic views of humanity. We should realize, though, that the particular view of humanity can have a major influence on our view of nursing.

2.2.2 Formulating a domain of nursing

Related to the dissatisfaction discussed above was, and is, the need to formulate what the specifics of nursing are. What is the domain of nursing? One important principle in this connection is that nursing has its own field, and cannot be reduced to one of the other scientific disciplines such as, for instance, medicine. We would also fail to do justice to the nursing discipline if we regarded it as a combination of extracts from several disciplines such as sociology, psychology, pharmacology and medicine. Within the profession there has been the need to describe the specific boundaries of nursing. Is a nurse simply a doctor's helper, or is there more to the profession?

Other disciplines also have their own specific problems demarcating their domain. Remedial education, for instance, has been through several changes. Initially it developed largely independent from educational science, and its orientation was strongly medical (van Gennep, 1988). It would be wrong, however, to assume that there can be rigid boundaries between any two related disciplines, as there will always be an overlap. The boundaries can change also over the years.

As we have seen, the boundaries of nursing have also changed. This becomes clear when we look at nursing education. From the beginning of this century, nursing education concentrated on medical knowledge. Within the context at the time, this was inevitable and understandable.

Now, though, nursing education draws its material from various disciplines including psychology, sociology, law, remedial education and so on. In a way this has been an important step forward, although it has led to a situation in which the field of nursing seems to be little more than a hotch-potch of various disciplines. It is not, of course, suggested that nursing should cease to examine and use the knowledge of other disciplines; simply that nursing theory development can help to clarify the domain of the discipline. This does not mean, though, that a simple statement about 'what nursing is really all about' will suffice.

Because nursing is interconnected with society (see also section 1.3), nursing as we know it today is a product of several factors. Financial factors, for instance, affect the boundaries of health care, and therefore also those of nursing. The strong emphasis on medical-technical factors in recent decades has also led to care, as such, taking a back seat. Nurses must take part of the blame for this. Emphasis has been placed on just giving the patient his or her medication, rather than on the personal attention which the nurse has the potential to give to the patient. In many cases, giving attention is at least as important as administering the prescribed medication.

There can be different ideas about what is meant by the 'domain' of nursing; it can be used to refer to the nursing field of duties, activity or knowledge. We lack the space here to take this any further.

2.2.3 The patient-centred approach
Another characteristic the different theories have in common is the more patient-centred approach, as opposed to the traditional functional ap-

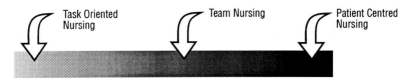

Figure 2.2 *Continuum of the orientation by which the nursing care is organized.*

proach of the nursing profession. A patient-centred approach is related both to how the care is organized, and to the nurse's attitude. We can distinguish between patient-centredness:

— as an *attitude* towards the patients (individually); and
— as a *form of organization* of the delivery of care within a ward, group or unit.

A more patient-centred organizational model can be a condition for this kind of attitude. Patient-centredness as an organizational principle is not sufficient to achieve patient-centredness as an attitude as well, although it will probably make some contribution to it!

Over the past few decades, there has been a move from task-oriented to patient-centred organizational principles for the delivery of nursing care. The two forms can be regarded as the two ends of a continuum, with a smooth transition; team nursing is somewhere in the middle (figure 2.2). One theory will be more concerned with patient-centredness than another. The *Integrating Nursing* theory, for instance, has worked out this principle in great detail. Assignment of patients to nurses during their admission is a key concept in this model. It is comparable to the principle of primary nursing, and that of the 'named nurse' (Marr & Giebing, 1994). But often, naturally, in the practical situation we come across mixed forms. Within a team, for instance, the work tends to be carried out in a rather task-oriented way. But it is also possible that the nursing of the team as a whole is carried out in a more patient-centred way, for instance in allocating rooms.

2.2.4 The nursing process
Many theories make use of the Nursing Process. For the last couple of years, the nursing process has been a generally accepted structure of nursing conduct. Although these theories differ in the number of stages and the contents of this process, they agree upon the general principles (Meleis, 1991). Some theorists hold, however, that use of the Nursing Process contradicts a holistic approach towards those in need of care.

2.2.5 Four core concepts

The last characteristic we want to mention here is that the various nursing theories share the following four core elements, or essential concepts (see among others, Fawcett 1989):

1 human being, person or patient
2 health; illness
3 environment
4 nursing.

It is generally thought that, in order to *be* a nursing theory, a theory should say something about these concepts and how they interrelate. These central elements are often referred to as the 'meta-paradigms'. This does not mean that these concepts are dealt with by theorists in separate sections. Usually, however, the reader needs to get the information from various places in the text.

A view of the human being normally goes hand in hand with a world view. Usually, both of these together also determine our view of health and disease (and of suffering, dying and death). Based on this is our view of nursing, treatment and recovery. In addition, the current theories usually indicate how these four concepts interrelate. If, for instance, nursing is only defined in terms of supporting the treatment of disease, there will be little attention paid by the nurses to preventative activities.

The choice of these four central elements and the term 'meta-paradigm' may be disputed (see, among others, Grypdonck 1991, Fawcett 1993). But, because there is a reasonable amount of consensus about these four concepts, we will use them in this book and in the evaluation instrument. In recent American meta-theoretical literature they are still mentioned (Marriner-Tomey 1989, Leddy & Pepper 1993, Wesley 1992, Fawcett 1993). In any case, it is relevant to look at these elements when comparing the different theories.

The theories often differ in the emphasis that is given to the different elements. Florence Nightingale, for instance, mainly emphasized the patient's environment, and paid little attention to the relationship between nurse and patient (see also the appendices).

2.3 Classifications

It is useful to make a brief remark here about the developments concerning classifications or taxonomies of nursing diagnoses and nursing interventions, such as those of the NANDA, Gordon, the NIC and others. Since 1990, attempts have also been made to formulate a uniform classification of nursing diagnoses and interventions for The Nether-lands as well. This is of great importance, as elementary concepts (such as 'sleeping problem', 'agitation', 'fatigue' and 'pain') are used in very different ways within the profession. Both the intra-disciplinary and the inter-disciplinary communication could be improved this way.

At present, the development and use of classification systems usually takes place separately from the development of theories (even though a few American theorists have been closely involved in developing classi-fication). We can compare this with two trails going in the same direction but apparently not touching each other. Through the development and spread of different classifications a confusing situation could arise.

An important difference between a classification system and a theory is that the first does not offer a general, interrelated unity, in spite of a few interrelated concepts within a classification. In a way, the development of a diagnosis could be regarded as developing theory on *micro-level* (or even sometimes *middle-range level*) as it is concerned with the description, explanation, prediction and/or prescription of separate phenomena. It is concerned with clarifying concepts (see also Meleis, 1991, p 160-2). A classification system which combines nursing diagnoses and interven-tions provides hardly any guidelines on which the *choice* of the most desirable kind of care in various situations can be based.

Diagnoses which are formulated in an objective way are also coloured by underlying views. The development of *both* theories and classifications are of importance to nursing, and I do not think that focusing on either of these exclusively will enhance the development of the profession.

2.4 Professional codes of conduct
Both nationally and internationally, various professional codes (such as the UKCC code of professional conduct) are in use. They state some of the basic principles for nursing conduct, including the nurse's attitude, and these are points about which there is a fair degree of consensus within nursing. Like the current nursing theories, they take responsibility for the nursing conduct, both internally and towards other carers and patients, and indicate minimum standards which can be expected. One important difference is that they contain a number of statements which do not clearly interrelate, are concise, and are of a very general character. They also have a strongly normative character and usually only state the minimum requirements. These codes fulfil a different, but important, function and we may expect nursing theories to be in accordance with their principles to a reasonable extent.

CHAPTER THREE

Types of Theories

There are all kinds of theories, and in the literature we come across several classifications of their different *types*. There is not always consensus about these classifications, but we want to discuss a few of the commonly used ones here as they are important for the evaluation of theories. In appendix 5, tables 5 to 9, some more classifications of types of theories are given, and these are based on the *contents* of the theories. The classifications in this chapter mainly relate to their form. We should not always have similar expectations from theories of different types, and this means that it is not always possible to compare them. This should be taken into account when theories are evaluated and applied. Usually, a theory does not fit entirely into a single category of these classifications: it often fulfils several of the functions at a time, with an emphasis on one of them. The theorist's own ideas about his or her theory can give us a useful insight, and we can also find out what other authors have said and take their impressions, as well as our own, into account.

3.1 Function

A theorist can have various *aims* with a theory, and it can relate to reality in different ways. The system used in this section can best be described as a classification according to function: what kind of function does the theory have? We usually distinguish four categories: descriptive, explanative, predictive and prescriptive, sometimes described as situation-changing or situation-producing (figure 3.1).

A theory's function, or aim, might be 'only' to describe existing phenomena, but it may also try to explain these phenomena. Theories with an essentially descriptive character take reality as their starting point. Virginia Henderson, for instance, originally gave a description of what she thought were the specifics of nursing. A prescriptive theory provides

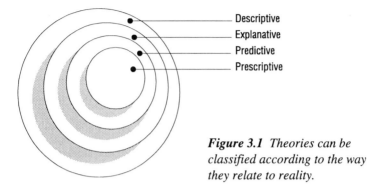

Descriptive
Explanative
Predictive
Prescriptive

Figure 3.1 *Theories can be classified according to the way they relate to reality.*

propositions aimed at changing the existing situation. It deals with the desirability of the situation and the way the patient is cared for, and questions what is important and what deserves priority. A theory which is (or aims to be) presciptive presupposes the other levels. To be able to prescribe, a theory also usually contains descriptions and explanations.

3.2 Level

Another classification which is used regularly in the literature is that of Dickoff and James (1968). A few authors hold that this one is similar to the one described above, while others regard it as consisting of the different stages of the development of theories — the authors themselves speak of different 'levels'. With regard to nursing, they give preference in the long term to developing theories of the fourth type, which are situation-producing. Theories of the fourth level have been developed in more detail than factor-isolating theories (figure 4).

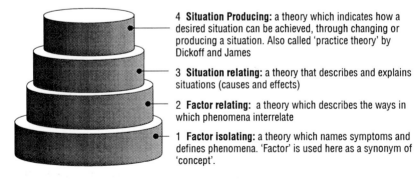

4 **Situation Producing:** a theory which indicates how a desired situation can be achieved, through changing or producing a situation. Also called 'practice theory' by Dickoff and James

3 **Situation relating:** a theory that describes and explains situations (causes and effects)

2 **Factor relating:** a theory which describes the ways in which phenomena interrelate

1 **Factor isolating:** a theory which names symptoms and defines phenomena. 'Factor' is used here as a synonym of 'concept'.

Figure 3.2 *Types of theories (according to Dickoff and James)*

Each higher level presupposes, and is based on, the preceding levels. According to Dickoff and James the theories of the first three levels are not yet full nursing theories, but they indicate what should be expected from such a theory (Dickoff, James & Wiedenbach, 1968). Dickoff and James hold that theories are not discovered, or derived from the practical situation, but invented for a certain purpose (Dickoff and James, 1968).

They feel that theories geared towards a practical discipline such as nursing should offer more than just a description or prediction of reality, and that a theory should also aim to help create reality and change it in a certain way. A theory, therefore, should contain both the final aim and the means of achieving this. Integrating Nursing is an example of a theory which aims to be situation-producing (and which is, therefore, also prescriptive).

Some authors equate Dickoff and James' classification with the classification according to range discussed in the section below. The two classifications are, however, of a different order.

3.3 Scope

Theories can have a different range or scope (which means that they cover different areas of reality). This is also often referred to as 'differences in levels of abstraction'. Usually the following distinction is made with regard to the scope of theories:

— *Micro-level theory* relates to a very small area of reality, one single phenomenon. It can relate, for instance, to one specific area of nursing care, like how to deal with decubitus. Sometimes we also speak of a 'practice-theory' or 'single-domain theory';
— *Middle-range theory* is concerned with a number of related phenomena. An example is Maslow's well-known theory about the hierarchy of needs;
— *Grand-theory* is the most abstract and wide-ranging type of theory, offering broad frameworks and a broad perspective. Many of the existing nursing theories have this range;
— *Meta-theory* is the theoretical consideration of theories and their development. It relates to philosophical principles or the method of developing theories (the epistemology).

Figure 3.3 and table 3.1 will help to clarify this classification.

In fact, no nursing theory exists at the meta-theory level. Following the analogy used in table 3.1, meta-theory level could be compared with cartography itself. Cartography is the study of how maps are made, but

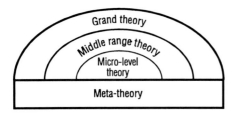

Figure 3.3 Theories classified according to their range. Meta-theory is, in fact, not a separate level but concerns the epistemology.

it is not a map itself. It formulates how good maps should be made and how they should be read. This book itself is actually concerned with the meta-theoretical level. In nursing, the meta-theory is still in its infancy. Every map is a scaled-down depiction of part of the real world. It can be filled with different kinds of detail, based on political boundaries, ethnic groups, languages, climate, gross national product, population density of the population, industrialization and so on. To follow our analogy, these could be nursing, medical, sociological or biological 'maps' or combinations of these.

This comparison makes it clear that the differences in scope do not exclude each other, but rather they assume each other. It also shows that each level necessarily involves a *reduction* of reality. No theory on its own offers a complete picture of reality, just as when you look at a map of the country you do not see the whole world. Nor do you see the different streets of any one town, let alone of all the towns. The 'ideal theory' should encompass all three different levels, or at least complement other theories of a similar, higher or lower level. The comparison with geographical boundaries shows that these lines are not fixed, they can move. Maps are only snapshots in time, outdated the moment they appear. Here again, our comparison with theories is relevant.

Current theories are usually in the range of grand-theory or middle-range theory, and the distinction between the two is not always clear-cut. There is still scope for differing opinions.

Table 3.1

Range	Comparison
Grand-theory	a broad theory which offers a complete survey of the reality of the nursing situation: can be compared with the map of a country
Middle-range theory	more specific, comparable to a county map. Covers an area with fairly clear boundaries
Micro-level	detailed, comparable to a town map

CHAPTER FOUR

The Importance
of Theories

What is the importance of theories and their development? In previous chapters, their usefulness has already been touched on. We will pursue this subject a bit further here, but for a more extensive discussion we refer the reader to the relevant literature. Within nursing, as in many other disciplines, we have 'theoretical pluralism': once we have come to recognize the importance of nursing theory in general, we will often wonder why there should be so many *different* ones. We will come back to this in section 4.2.

4.1 The functions of theories

Firstly, it should be made clear that theories are a *means* to achieve an end, rather than an end in themselves. A theory is normally not meant to be a static product. Theory development is a cyclic, continuous and dynamic process (Meleis 1991) and one which requires time. Theories and their usefulness should not, therefore, be assessed only on what we see in the practical situation at a given moment. We must also consider any future possibilities, and this means that each sector within the profession should try out theories intensively. Amongst other factors, the usefulness of a theory depends on what we aim to achieve with it and on its level and range (see chapter three). The ultimate importance of a theory is determined by how others use it — in, for instance, research or nursing practice. A good theory which stays unused is probably worth less than a poor theory which is applied in practice. Depending on various factors including their stage of development, their level and their aims or functions, theories can be useful in one or more of the following ways.

1. As a frame of reference

A nursing theory functions as a frame of reference or as a pattern of thought. It helps to formulate the boundaries of the nursing domain and enable us to look at the specifics of nursing. A pattern of thought can be likened to a picture frame, holding what the theorist concerned believes to be the nursing domain. It can indicate both to the nursing profession and to the outside world what nursing is, and is not, about.

2. To order phenomena
By interrelating phenomena, a meaningful unity can be formed. The fact is that reality is very complex, and this is true of the everyday reality of nursing. Theories can arrange this reality in a certain order, although this simplifies reality. Consider the following example concerning a phenomenon very well-known to nurses. Patients develop wounds in different places. On closer examination, it appears that the wounds occur mainly in bedridden patients. Various factors appear to be interrelated: for instance, the wounds are always preceded by red areas on the skin. Arranging phenomena in this way can guide our thinking, observation and interpretation, enabling the nurse to observe more purposefully. Some red areas on the skin can now be interpreted as the beginning of decubitus, and steps can be taken to deal with the problem in a goal-oriented way.

3. To give direction in the practical situation
A theory can give direction to the practice of nursing care, and have a supportive function in nursing administration. According to Grypdonck (1991), a particular view will give direction in the practical situation once individual nurses have familiarized themselves with it and studied it in detail. A theory can help when choices have to be made, when for instance the priorities of the nursing care need to be determined. Nursing theories can be used to motivate the nurse's thinking and conduct, and to account for this conduct to other disciplines, potential care seekers, insurers and the government. Thus, nursing theories can also have an influence at the macro-level.

4. As the basis of nursing education
A grand-theory or middle-range theory can be used as a framework for education, giving structure to and determine the contents of a curriculum. Micro-level theories can, because of their more concrete character, be used directly in nursing practice and for discussion during classes. A few nursing theories were initially designed not as 'theories' but as part of the curriculum of a certain training course.

5. As a framework for nursing research
A theory can give direction to research and prevent it from remaining restricted to isolated data. Statements in a theory should possibly lead to

presuppositions which can be tested: these are called *hypotheses*. Theories should be potentially testable (see also section 5.4).

6. As the basis of nursing ethics

A theory can also function as the basis for the ethics of nursing conduct. At present, there is a tendency to give a broader meaning to ethics than simply the boundaries of what is permissible and what is not.

7. As the basis for quality assurance

The quality of nursing care can be assessed using a theory to provide criteria or standards. When a theory describes the care that is desirable or necessary, the actual care delivered can be evaluated using the theory as the standard against which it can be measured.

The usefulness of theory development (process) rests on the usefulness of the theories (product) as such. In other words, as long as nursing theories are useful, theory development will be useful as well.

4.2 Theoretical pluralism

Within nursing we find 'theoretical pluralism', which means that different, conflicting, and partly overlapping theories are influential at the same time within the discipline. This diversity may create confusion, but it also offers opportunities for theories to develop from different perspectives (this also occurs within other scientific disciplines). The calls for a single comprehensive '*super theory*' of nursing seem to have ceased. Evers states: 'The complexity and variety of nursing processes also show that we need a number of different theories. It is an illusion to think that one day the one and only nursing theory will be invented. The object of the practice of nursing is so complex that theoretical pluralism is essential' (Evers 1991).

Grypdonck (1981) expands on the underlying epistemological view that there should really only be a single nursing theory. Repeated reference is made to the ideas of the physicist Thomas Kuhn and his 'Structure of Scientific Revolutions'. According to Kuhn, if a discipline has different, co-existing theories we cannot speak of it as a science. At that point, the discipline is at a pre-scientific ('pre-paradigmatic') stage. Grypdonck holds that this boundary between science and pre-science is largely *arbitrary*.

Kuhn has made this idea into a basic rule of science (ibid). In other words, Kuhn's definition of science has acquired a strongly normative character. According to Grypdonck, the desirability and development of a science as Kuhn sees it requires further research. A third objection in referring to Kuhn's paradigm in regard to the development of the discipline of nursing science is concerned with the particular exceptions Kuhn made for medicine, law and applied science; those disciplines that owe their existence mainly to fulfilling external social needs. Grypdonck questions, therefore, whether nursing is at all suitable for paradigmatic development. A comparison with medicine shows that the reply to this question would be a negative one (ibid). She states, on the other hand, that '...theoretical pluralism is important for science in general, and could even be one of the *strong points* of the social sciences, and should therefore certainly not be opposed...', and this view is supported by several other authors (Grypdonck, 1981, italics GHH).

Although the relationships between different theories and the 'boundary' between what is science and what is not are important points of discussion for the scientific foundations of nursing, we will not pursue this any further here. It is a comforting thought, though, that disciplines such as medicine, sociology and psychology do not comply with Kuhn's criteria either.

Whether a theory can be used in a satisfactory way in the practical nursing care situation, in administration or in education depends on various factors. One of these concerns the profession itself. Not everyone in nursing is convinced of the importance of having our own theories, and to some extent a critical attitude from the practical side of the profession is a positive thing.

However, we should face the alternative: the consequence of rejecting nursing theories is that nursing practice will continue to be based on tradition, authority, ritual and similar forces, or else it will have to stay mainly dependent upon theories from various other disciplines. Optimizing relations between the different elements of the nursing profession, and stressing the distinctive features of the profession, will stimulate further development — especially when the development and the use of theories are concerned.

We should be aware that when a theory 'does not work in practice', this can be due to factors within the theory, to factors within the practical situation, or to both. It is important that the causes for these problems are traced and solutions sought. Complaints from nurses that 'theories are *just* theories, and they are bound to fail in the practical situation anyway' are unfounded, narrow-minded, and an obstruction to the further development of nursing into a serious profession. Yet, the desire for simplicity and unambiguity within nursing is understandable.

A sound foundation for nursing, based on theories and research, is of the utmost importance in giving the discipline a clear, accountable position. Nurses must be able to explain *what* they do, *how* they do it, and *why* they do it. In other words, it is not only the 'doing', but also the 'thinking' that counts. In this respect nursing is well behind other disciplines, and this is a problem that should be dealt with.

Why not look at it from a different angle: Kurt Lewin, the German-American psychologist (quoted by Madsen, 1975) said that:

> *'Nothing is as practical as a good theory'*,

and as Blok has pointed out:

> *'Columbus did not travel around aimlessly. He sailed to the West on the basis of a plausible theory.'*

CHAPTER FIVE

The Application of Theories

In America as well as in Europe attempts have already been made to use nursing theories in the practical situation. In this chapter, we will look at how the theories are used today in education, administration and nursing practice. We will have to pay attention especially to the *opportunities* for using theories which can be attained once problems such as unfamiliarity with theories have been dealt with. In general, we should not expect more from a theory than it aims to achieve (just as you cannot make a delicate picture frame with a large sledgehammer or saw thick wooden planks with a kitchen knife). This means that a theory should always be considered within its own particular context. As we have seen, the usefulness of a theory is ultimately determined by what others, in administration or research for instance, actually do with it.

5.1 Administration

Within nursing administration the need to make principles or views more explicit at an institutional and/or team level, has grown with the desire to decide upon and state a nursing *policy*, which may in turn be based on a specific nursing theory. This can have a motivating effect on nurses. It can be used for arranging the various tasks and the responsibilities within a unit. Patient-centred nursing, for instance, can only take place when it is initiated, guided and carried by the policy. A theory can also offer a broad framework for policy with regard to the quality of care, allowing standards and criteria to be formulated.

Sometimes, the use of a theory is limited to the introduction of a few tangible organizational principles taken from the theory. Such organizational elements are usually the more concrete parts. It may be, for instance, that an organization introduces a form for the assessment of nursing history based on Roper's '12 Activities of Daily Living' and then believe they are working 'according to Roper'. Likewise, the introduction of Integrated Nursing can be limited to the allocation of nurses to certain patients, while no attention is paid to the basic scientific nursing attitude the theory propounds, the patient is not approached holistically, or the head nurse sticks to her traditional role.

Professional guidance is essential when a particular theory is being introduced into an organization, with regard to both its content and the process of application. Making a choice from the theories available requires a lot of preparation; and an instrument of evaluation like the one presented in this book can be helpful. Extra training also plays an important role, and the instrument of evaluation can be useful here as well. In general, processes of change are very intensive and require a lot of preparation, clarification and consultation. Working on the basis of a particular theory can also involve a *cultural change* in an organisation. This all means that the pros and cons need to be balanced against each other carefully. We will not discuss processes of change any further here, as there are many publications which deal with it.

It is strongly recommended that a *data-bank* containing all the relevant, up-to-date documents concerned with a chosen theory, is kept at a central place within the organization. The specialist journals regularly contain articles about the different theories, and summaries of their main points can be distributed throughout the departments or units involved.

5.2 Nursing practice
In certain conditions, particularly when the administration's policy is conducive to such a development, a theory can take shape in practice. The application of theories in the practical situation of nursing care and administration is still in its infancy, partly as a result of factors within practice (unfamiliarity with the theories) and partly due to factors related to theory development itself (abstraction). Much has been (and will be) written about how to link 'theory' and 'practice'. As nurses acquire greater amounts of knowledge about theories, either through education or refresher courses, the theories will gradually have greater conse-quences for the profession at the practical caring level. As we have said before, a particular theory or view will actually give direction in nursing practice once the nurses become familiar with it (see section 4.1).

Not every theory requires organizational changes. Although within a single team or unit preference should usually be given to working from the same theory, there are also theories which concentrate mainly on the nurse's personal attitude. As an individual, the nurse can choose to base her work on Christian principles, for instance, or on van der Bruggen's anthropological views of nursing. It would probably be more difficult if an individual nurse decided to work from an anthroposophical angle, as this requires specific changes in the environment because the environment in which caring takes place plays an essential therapeutic role in this theory, and interventions not commonly used in health care might be chosen.

One example of a model which is presently used in various institutions, both in general nursing and psychiatric nursing, is Integrated Nursing (Koene, Grypdonck, Rodenbach and Windey, 1989). This model has consequences for higher and intermediate levels of management as well as for nursing care. Its aim is to reorientate nursing.

Evaluating theories using a suitable instrument can stimulate the team or the individual nurses to think more deeply about their own profession. Discussing a theory during a team meeting can be a very interesting experience. Theories can also be introduced during clinical lessons[1], thus contributing to the development of the professionalism of each individual nurse.

5.3 Education
Nursing research has become a fairly well established element at nursing training colleges. The situation regarding the development and use of nursing theories is less clear. Research, after all, is rather more practical and this apparently makes it easier to argue for its importance. Yet there is an increasing number of text books which are based on a particular nursing theory. These books are in part a further development, realization or interpretation of the theories. But how else are the theories used?

Grypdonck (1991) concludes, after visiting several colleges in the Netherlands at baccalaureate level, that two different patterns can be distinguished. On the one hand there are those colleges which have decided to give predominance to one single theory. The students work with or from that theory, course readers are based on it, and when the student is doing a work placement the theory is applied. In that case, the student becomes acquainted with other theories at a later stage. One problem of this approach is that the student may learn to adapt reality to the theory, as not all theories are applicable in all practical situations. On the other

---

1 Clinical lessons are a kind of team meetings in a ward or unit where nurses can exchange ideas and discuss recent developments in nursing or medicine. Once or twice a month one of the nurses or students can introduce a particular topic.

hand, there are training colleges which do not choose one particular theory, but work with various different ones. The students learn to apply different theories to a caring situation, sometimes making their own choice of which theory they want to use. Grypdonck herself gives preference to a third possibility, which is the discussion of themes which are (or should be) dealt with in a theory. This means that students are trained in a more flexible way, and learn to comment on theories and make suggestions for improvements. In other words, they will become more actively involved. Thus, students will find it easier to deal with the different views they come across within the different organizations for which they work. Another point to make is that theory development is an ongoing development and it is likely that after a few years new insights will become prevalent. Working with an instrument of evaluation will presumably fit in well with this third approach.

It is necessary within education to clarify theories and the process of theory development. Use of an evaluation instrument like the one presented here can help to give insight into the different theories, making it easier to work with them both in education and in practice. This applies to tutors and students alike, and is necessary because the subject matter is complex and relatively unfamiliar. Our knowledge about the different theories can be increased in this way. Also, when the different views and theories of the supportive subjects from other disciplines are the only or the main ones used, the students can get too fragmentary a picture of nursing. A theory (or more than one theory) can be used as a backbone for the entire nursing curriculum.

As education is such a crucial issue, we will pay special attention to the relationship between theories and education in this section. In training, the student nurse acquires the basic tools she needs to carry out her work. The ability to evaluate is also essential for a well-argued final project and for the ability to form and argue for a point of view about the nursing profession. To higher education students evaluation has another, more direct, importance: by evaluating theories they will develop a *skill* which will enable them to study theories and work with their practical applica-tion. The student learns how to look at and think systematically about theories and their practical implications. Having looked at theories in a structured way they can contribute to discussion about the use of theories within the institution where they work, or offer theoretical insights into the practical situation. They could, for instance, give clinical lessons or start a study group. Their background will enable them to discuss a theory critically when it is under consideration, and thus might make it possible to prevent the application of a theory being restricted to a number of organizational principles while the institution and the nurses believe they are putting a theory into practice (as noted above). Thus, education can fulfil an important function in promoting the adequate use of nursing theories in the nursing field. It is to be hoped that this will lead to more justice being done to the intentions of a theorist than is the case when only a few random concepts or some single part from a theory are used.

Students can also be offered the opportunity to make an in-depth study of one particular theory for their *final project*, and the evaluation instrument presented in this book can be used for this purpose. They can, for instance, pay extra attention to the extent to which the theory can be applied in practice. By interviewing nurses in places where a specific theory is applied they can also gain some insight into how others who work with the theory feel about it.

Attention should also be paid to the link between theories and the student's *work placement*. By working through a few assignments which deal with nursing theories, the integration between theory and practice can be encouraged. Such an assignment might involve, for instance, asking the students to make a nursing plan in practice based on the theory they have studied.

Another problem which occurs at nursing colleges is that of *integrating* nursing theories into the whole of the curriculum, especially where the tutors concerned are not nurses. The views of the various theorists could be discussed at different stages during the course—when we are dealing with prevention or patient education, for instance, reference could be made to nursing theories. When psychiatry is dealt with we could quote what anthroposophic nursing says about the subject, or refer to Peplau or Roy. When we are discussing philosophical and ideological questions, nursing theories could be placed in a wider perspective. One example of a philosophical school is existentialism, to which anthropologic nursing and other theories are related.

Tutors, both of nursing and of other disciplines, could use the evaluation instrument to work through one or more theories in small groups. This could be extended, increasing the tutors' knowledge of the theories and generally contributing to a more integrated role for nursing theories within the curriculum as a whole. Nursing theories will then no longer be an *isolated* subject. Thinking about nursing and themes relevant to nursing could thus be promoted.

To make searches of the professional literature easier, it is desirable that all of the documentation of journal articles about different theories is organized at a central place. The library seems the obvious choice. It must also have a good collection of both primary literature (that is, papers written by the actual theorist) and secondary literature (commentaries by others). Books about the development of theories (meta-theory) and nursing research should also be available, to the tutors at the very least.

It would be beneficial to have nursing literature files such as the INI[1] or CINAHL[2] and Medline[3] available on CD-ROM. It is also necessary to enrich the library with a few leading specialist journals like *Nursing Research* and the *Journal of Advanced Nursing* if these are not already available within the college (see also the comments in appendix 6).

5.4 Research

As we have seen, theory development and research can be regarded as instruments of science. Ideally, they complement each other and interact with each other (we mentioned this briefly in section 4.1). Broadly speaking, there are three ways in which they relate to each other in a practical science like nursing:

1 Theories can offer a *framework* for nursing research. They can bring a focus to research, and prevent it being restricted to isolated data. We can make a further classification here:
   a. a theory may be referred to during the initial phases of research; to be used as a point of departure; *or*
   b a theory may be referred to after the research has been carried out. After completion of the research an attempt is made to fit the results to a particular theory. Although this will not be the primary aim of the research, it may contribute indirectly to the development of a theory.
2. Research can also be used to *test* the statements or propositions made in a theory. It should be possible to derive hypotheses from these statements, and theories ought to be testable. A theory can thus be based on empirical data, acquiring a more scientific char-

---

1 *International Nursing Index*, a traditional literature file with titles and keywords, in book form.
2 *Cumulative Index of Nursing and Allied Health Literature*, an index of nursing literature on CD-ROM. It also contains literature from related disciplines.
3 *Medline* is the CD-ROM version of the *Index Medicus*, and it also contains international literature in languages other than English. It includes literature from related disciplines.

Table 5.1 Possible relationships between theories and research (a dynamic and ideally cyclic process).

Starting point	Next step	Possible conitinuation
1a Theory (framework → Research → as starting point)		Adjusted theory
1b Research →	Theory (as framework afterwards)	
2 Theory →	Research (to test → theory)	Theory adjusted or rejected
3 Research (or → research projects)	Theory →	Further research (types 1a or 2)

acter. It can also occur, however, that as a result of testing, the theory as a whole or parts of it need to be adjusted or rejected. In future more importance should be given to testing theories through research, with the aim of further developing nursing science. Testing through research is especially suitable for theories within the micro- or middle-range levels. A grand-theory as a whole cannot be tested directly because of its global character nor is it possible to test all its different, separate, statements and assumptions.

3 Lastly, research may lead to the development of theories. On the basis of one or more research projects, a new theory can be developed, and this theory will thus be based on research done in the practical field. A series of research projects on, for instance, the subject of pain, can lead to a nursing theory about pain. On the basis of this new theory, further research can be done.

Table 5.1 shows the relation between theories and research.

On the basis of the analysis of a number of research articles, Jaarsma and Dassen (1993) give an overview of the use of theories in research. This overview also shows the different roles theories can fulfil with regard to research, and the role research can play in theory development.

Nursing research ought to act in service of the development of nursing theory. Knowledge acquired through research contributes to the knowledge described in theories, and the theories hold and give structure to the knowledge on which nursing science is based. As this relationship lies mainly in the field of science, we will not discuss this any further here: the interested reader can find ample literature elsewhere (including Meleis 1991, Polit & Hungler 1991 and Fawcett & Downs 1986).

CHAPTER SIX

Considerations in Applying Theories

As we have seen in the previous chapter, theories are gradually being used throughout the different elements of the nursing profession. In this chapter we will discuss some of the points which influence the use of theories. There is, for instance, a gap between theory and practice, and for a fruitful discussion about the use of theories it is useful to look at this gap critically. We will then examine the choice of a theory, and finally we will discuss the extent to which a theory can be introduced in a practical situation.

6.1 The gap between theory and practice

There is, undeniably, a *gap* between theory and practice, in nursing just as in other disciplines. To be able to bridge this gap (or rather these gaps) we first need to know exactly what they consist of and where they are. Often the problems are dismissed by a statement that we are dealing with the difference between the *real* world and an *ideal* one. Reality is 'just the way things happen to be', and the ideal is 'utopian, nicely formulated, but completely unachievable'. At this point the discussion usually ends, leaving the participants (and the issues) no further forward.

It is a useful first step to clarify what is meant by 'theory' and 'practice'. We have a 'practice' of caring, and we have theoretical views. But THE theory does not exist, and neither does THE practical situation. Part of the gap between 'theory' and 'practice' is therefore fictitious, based on timidity and an improper division between 'acting' and 'thinking' (figure 6.1).

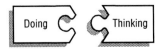

Doing ⊃⊂ Thinking

Figure 6.1 The gap between acting and thinking.

Thus, the impression is given that we need to make a choice between thinking and acting, and in practice the emphasis is on the acting. Nursing, however, requires that people both act *and* think thoroughly about what they do. We must also remember that our thinking affects our acting both consciously or subconsciously. Our feelings about a subject have consequences for our actions and the choices we make. To promote a well considered way of providing care it is necessary that nurses develop the habit of thinking thoroughly about the factors which influence their actions, including the desirable outcomes, priorities and consequences of their interventions.

A more fruitful discussion, and one which will probably bring less frustration, can be achieved when the gap between theory and practice is regarded as a difference between *reality* and *desirability*. Formulating a desirable situation (as many theories do) does not mean that this can become reality overnight: there is usually a long road from desirability to reality. However, when we compare the current situation with that of ten to thirty years ago, it becomes obvious that change is definitely possible in nursing (figure 6.2).

It appears, therefore, that the gap between reality and desirability is often dependent on time and/or place. What is still an ideal in one situation, has often become reality in another (consider, for instance, the use of nursing care plans or the introduction of patient-centred nursing). When we look at the reasons why the desirable situation has become reality in one particular situation we will find that the gap is to some extent 'culture-dependent'. Often, within a single organization one ward can work with nursing plans successfully while another department does not succeed in working with them at all. In such a situation, it is impossible to explain the discrepancy on the basis of objective differences between departments. Critical analysis will often show that the 'culture' of the different wards plays an important part. The *attitude* of individual nurses or of a team can have a strongly negative influence on the processes of change.

As we have seen, practical care and nursing science share the same principal objective — the 'satisfactory delivery of care'. Yet, there are a number of substantial differences between 'theory' (and science in

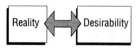

Figure 6.2 *An actual gap might exist between the desirable situation and reality. This gap can be bridged, but only by deliberate, external action.*

general) on the one hand, and 'practice' on the other. Some of these are as follows.

— Theories and research in general aim to objectify: to acquire *general* knowledge by asking questions such as:
  – 'What eating problems do mentally handicapped people have? How can these be adequately prevented or dealt with?'
  – 'What problems are experienced by patients who need a rest-cure because of a slipped disc?'
— In nursing practice we deal with the *individual* patient, with his own subjective perception and circumstances. We look for knowledge about *this* person in this specific situation. In other words, it is aimed at concrete situations. We might ask, for example:
  –'What eating problems does Hannah have? What therefore is the best way of stimulating her to eat?'
  – 'What problems does Mr Johnstone have as a result of his rest-cure? What is painful to him, and how can I help to alleviate the pain?'

A professional nurse must be able to use the general knowledge, combined with her personal experience, in the specific situation of the individual patient she is caring for. It is neither sufficient nor professional to apply knowledge from research or from a theory without adapting it consciously to a specific situation. Thus, the nurse's professional accountability is increased, and the quality of the nursing care will improve.

6.2 The choice of a theory

We will briefly discuss the choice of a theory. This can be influenced by many different factors, and must be done carefully, especially when the theory is being chosen within an organization or a team (though nurses can use a theory, or ideas derived from a theory, in their individual work as well). The choice of a theory for research work depends on different considerations. Based on her experience over a period of 25 years and on her discussions with students, scientists, nurses and managers in the United States and elsewhere, Meleis (1991) has listed a number of criteria which form the basis for these choices.

— *Personal:* Individuals who use this criterion discuss their personal comfort in using the theory, their intuitive choices, and theory's congruency with their philosophical view of life;
— *Mentor:* There are those who use a theory because they were mentored by a theorist. They spoke of personal influence, respect, personal contact and educational experience.

— *Theorist:* Who the theorists are, their standing in the field, their status and how well they are recognised were among the reasons that a theory was selected.

— *Literature support:* Others identified the availablility of extensive writings about the theory that gave them assurance of the level of significance of the theory and the status it holds.

— *Sociopolitical congruency:* The congruency between the theory implementation process and the sociopolitical as well as economic climate was another criterion often identified by audiences. These people spoke of a climate that supports one theory over another because, for example, it did not necessitate structural changes, it required minimal preparation, or it was imposed by administration.

— *Utility:* The ease with which the theory was understood and applied prompted a group of users to select a certain theory over another.

Meleis emphasizes these personal factors as influences on the decision to use a theory. She stresses that both objective and subjective processes can play a part in selection, and believes both are equally important to take into consideration. It is neither strange nor undesirable that subjective factors have an influence on the decision made, especially when the theory has a more abstract character, describing a certain viewpoint.

In practice, we see occasionally that the choice is not of a single, specific theory. Different reasons may be given for this, not all of which will be well thought out. An objection to using more than one theory is that the nursing practice may then become eclectic in character, with parts of different theories being used together in an arbitrary way. This can easily result in sort of hotch-potch of theories: consider, for example, a combination of Roper's 12 Activities of Daily Living with Roy's nursing process and Leininger's 'Sunrise Model'. This will seldom do justice to the theories involved. Yet the extent to which the user has the freedom to do this is an important and interesting point for discussion, and we return to it in the following chapter.

Systematic evaluation is an important aid to the choice of a theory. In chapter seven we will also discuss some important aspects of this.

6.3 Stages of application

Usually, once a theory has been chosen it cannot simply be stuck on to the practical situation. In addition to choosing the specific theory, we must also therefore decide on the *extent* to which we want to implement it. A theory can be introduced into the caring situation in different *stages*. While these are not absolute stages with clearly defined boundaries, they can give an impression of the degree to which the theory is applied in practice.

1 *Heard of* — we have heard of the theory, but do not consciously use it in any way.
2 *Familiarity with* — we are familiar with some of the ideas of a theory and conscious of the theory as a whole but do not yet apply it in any sort of practical sense. From reading or hearing about the theory we have become aware, for instance, of the importance of paying attention to the patient's environment.
3 *Partial use* — parts of the theory are used, or the theory is used occasionally. For instance, Orem's classification of self-care is used for taking histories, or a number of organizational principles from Integrated Nursing are introduced.
4 *Optimum usage* — at this stage, all or nearly all of the theory is used within a team or organization as a framework for the conduct of nursing, and it gives real direction to the nursing practice. It is unlikely that at the moment many theories are used at this stage. Further research will be needed to decide whether this is a desirable and feasible outcome.

There are also individual nurses who would like to base their work on a certain theory, but who do not receive any support from the team or the organization. Of course, the extent to which the theory can be used depends largely on the type of theory in question, but we will not find out what this extent is until we actually try it out. It will be obvious that the thorough *evaluation* of a theory is a prerequisite for its optimum usage, and this is the subject of the following chapter.

CHAPTER SEVEN

The Evaluation of Theories

So far, we have looked at the function of theorizing within nursing as a whole, and discussed the importance and application of theories. Yet the main aim of this book is to assist with the *evaluation* of nursing theories. With this in mind, we will first outline the main areas of evaluation and then discuss a few specific points. The Vijverberg Evaluation Instrument for Nursing Theories (the ENT) is based on these points, so the comments made in this chapter are also comments on the evaluation instrument. But before we do this, we will examine the usefulness of evaluating theories.

7.1 The usefulness of evaluation

Following Meleis (1991) we have chosen the term 'evaluation' because it has a more neutral meaning than a word like 'judgement', and we can distinguish various elements in evaluation, including description, analysis and criticism. Testing theories through research can also be part of the process of evaluation. There are several reasons we could give for evaluating theories, and we will discuss a few of them here. The relevant literature gives a more thorough treament of the subject. Depending on what we aim to achieve through evaluation and the points we choose to evaluate, the process can be useful for the following reasons:

1 Evaluation is particularly important for increasing our *knowledge* of and *insight* into a particular theory. An 'evaluation instrument' which gives a list of specific points is an aid to collecting this knowledge in a structured way. As the list has been made beforehand, its use will help to decrease subjectivity in the assessment.

2 Evaluation will reveal the major features of a theory; knowledge and insight will clarify its *aims*.

3 Evaluation can be used to look at the different *concepts* which are employed. Have they been used clearly and consistently?

4 The analysis of a theory can reveal implicit *presuppositions* and enable assessment of the logic used.

5 By enabling a theory's *usefulness* to be gauged, points 1 – 4 above make it easier to promote its application in nursing care, education, administration and research.

6 Theories can be *compared* with each other once they have been evaluated. The insights gained through evaluation make it possible to place theories side by side and compare them in a structured way. We can look at similarities and differences with regard to the criteria we select, and the stronger and weaker points of each theory can be found.

7.2 The main points of an evaluation

In order to make the evaluation of theories seem rather less abstract, it may be useful to make a comparison with the valuation of real estate.

A chartered surveyor will take three main areas into account. The first area is the *building* itself, its purpose and form. Are there sufficient windows? What about maintenance? What materials are used in the construction? The interior is also important. How many rooms are there, and are they appropriate to the building's purpose? A private house, for instance, will need a bathroom and a kitchen. The second area is concerned with *comfort*. Does the house only have a shower, or has it a bath as well? Has the kitchen been fitted recently, and is the space used in a convenient way? How big is the living-room? Where is the house situated, does it have nice views? The third area concerns the building's *foundations*: are they strong enough?

It will be clear that these three areas are interrelated. We should also, therefore, look at the *ways* in which they interconnect. Is the building

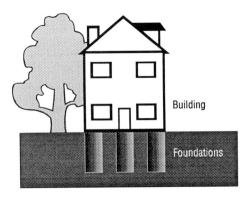

Figure 7.1 A nursing theory can be compared with a building. It has foundations and it can be used for different purposes. A surveyor will base his valuation on the building itself, its foundations and its suitability for various uses.

suitable for its purpose? Can it be easily adjusted to serve a different purpose if that is what the future occupier wants? The kind of building it is determines how the three areas are judged. Our expectations for a factory differ from those we will have of an office or a hospital. The degree of comfort within a building is slightly more subjective: one person's comfort may be another's source of annoyance. A surveyor will take this into account in his valuation, but the price will ultimately be determined by what the buyer is prepared to pay.

A building's comfort and the purposes which it can be used for are not determined solely by the building itself. It may be multi-functional by design, but inventive architecture can convert a factory into beautiful flats. Likewise, an individual can adapt a building to suit his own ideas about comfort. In table 7.1 a comparison is made between the valuation of buildings and the evaluation of nursing theories.

I propose to group the evaluation of theories into three areas similar to those shown in the table. The first area deals with principles and assumptions: we could call it the foundation of the theory. Theories do not float around in a vacuum. They are usually based on other ideas or theories. Their assumptions may be of a philosophical, ideological or religious nature, for instance, and can be generally accepted within society or within certain sectors of society. They may be formulated or stated *explicitly* by the theorist, but often they are made *implicitly*. The fact that a theory does not contain any explicit assumptions does not necessarily mean that it is of a more 'neutral' character or is actually based on fewer assumptions.

We should also note the extent to which the three main areas of a theory interact with each other. A theory can be based on very explicit principles which do not necessarily have any practical consequences. The view of the human being in van den Brink-Tjebbes' 'Nursing in respect of the

Table 7.1 *A comparison between the valuation of real estate and the evaluation of nursing theories.*

The valuation of real estate	The evaluation of nursing theories
foundation	underlying presuppositions, assumptions, and principles
building	the theory (content and form)
how the building can be used	its practical consequences and usefulness

higher rules pertaining to nursing' is explicitly rooted in Jewish and Christian principles which have been and are an essential part of our culture. Van den Brink-Tjebbes states, though, that one does not necessarily need to share these views personally to be able to use her theory.

It is possible that there is no logical cohesion between the three areas. Figures 7.2 to 7.5 show in a schematic way how the assumptions which are at the basis of a theory (A), the content of the theory itself (T) and the practical consequences of A and T (C) might interrelate. Several combinations are possible. The degree of overlap reflects the extent to which the main points are connected with one another. We would encourage the reader to bear this in mind when studying a theory, to try to form an idea of the cohesion built into it.

When a theory is evaluated, we should remember that the principles of the person carrying out the evaluation will, either consciously or subconsciously, affect the outcome. With most types of theories, this does not present a problem: it is acceptable for personal, subjective factors to

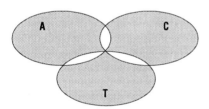

Figure 7.2 *The theory, its assumptions and its practical consequences hardly interrelate at all.*

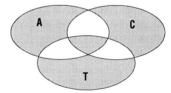

Figure 7.3 *In the ideal situation, there is a firm relationship between the theory, its principles and its practical consequences.*

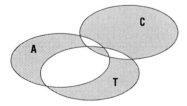

Figure 7.4 *The theory is firmly rooted in its assumptions, but these have hardly any practical consequences.*

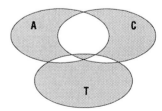

Figure 7.5 *The assumptions have practical consequences, but these are hardly related to the theory itself.*

influence the choice of a theory for use in nursing practice. Once again we can draw a parallel with house valuation. The user of a theory can decide to use only part of the theory, just as the user of a building can choose to use only part of the building. These personal factors should be paid attention to explicitly, as they do in practice partly determine the choice of the theory. Both objective and subjective processes are at work (see also sections 6.2 and 6.3).

In addition to the three main points, there are also a number of more general issues which affect evaluation. One such issue is a description of the theorists themselves. Other general questions might include, for instance, the reason why a theory has been developed, and the way in which it has been developed. These general points, which tend to be concerned with the theory's background, help to give an idea of the theory's context.

7.3 Evaluation points

As we have seen, it is important to evaluate theories adequately in order to gain insight into their differences and do justice to the intentions of the theorists. A theory can be evaluated in different ways and using different points of evaluation. Within nursing science there are some intruments of analysis already in use (see appendix 2), so it was neither desirable nor necessary for us to re-invent the wheel.

Some aspects of evaluation, however, are also outwith the scope of professional nursing education and the direct practice of nursing care. For this reason, we will not discuss evaluation through *testing* here, as this is usually done at a scientific level. There is, however, an important task here for nursing science: some of the points of evaluation deserve to be investigated at university level. The points discussed in this section are those which will be useful and meaningful within education and nursing practice. They are relevant to current nursing theories, most of which are at the range of grand-theory.

We have seen how evaluation can be divided roughly into three main areas. To prevent the construction of the evaluation instrument from becoming too artificial, these main areas are not separated in a rigid manner. There is a degree of overlap between some of them. Yet they do reflect the basic idea of starting from a few general aspects and finishing with the practical application of the theory. A short explanation or an example is given as clarification of each point, but the previous chapters will also help towards explanation. The numbering reflects the numbering of the Vijverberg evaluation instrument.

1. The theorist

To get a more complete view of a theory, it is useful to learn something about the theorists who developed it. What training do they have? In what fields do they work? How has their work developed? This will give an impression of the theorist's frame of reference, and help to paint a picture of the people behind the theory.

Information about this can often be found in the primary literature[1]. A number of meta-theorists also give us this kind of information, sometimes even including an address and a photograph (Marriner-Tomey, for instance). Students and nurses do not always realize, for instance, that American professors of nursing science and theorists are mainly women. Male nurses are less common there than in the Netherlands. This kind of background information will, for example, prevent you from speaking of 'his' theory when you are discussing the work of a female theoretician, like Roy.

2. The aim of the theory, or the reason why it has been formulated

This will give us greater insight into the background, the context and the intentions of the theory.

Some theorists did not set out to formulate a theory in the narrow sense (Marriner-Tomey 1989) but rather intended to provide a curriculum for nursing education.

3. The development of the theory

Theories differ considerably in the ways in which they developed. Some are one-off presentations, while others are adapted and refined over many years.

When we have a revised edition of a theory, we can check the publication dates of previous editions, and we can find out whether there are different prefaces to the different editions in the book (table 1 of appendix 5 can also be helpful in this respect). We can often find in this way whether the theory has been revised following research, practical experience or criticism, and we should pay close attention to any alterations. Van den Brink-Tjebbes, for instance, has altered the terminology she uses; she now speaks of 'human life care' rather than 'self-care', because the latter term caused confusion, for instance with Orem's interpretation of self-care.

---

1 In this context, primary literature refers to material written directly by the theoritician, while secondary literature refers to material written about the theory or the theoritician by others.

King has added a number of concepts to her theory in her latest book (King 1981). Leininger has altered some elements of her 'Sunrise Model' (Leininger 1991), although we should note that she did not make any significant alterations to her ideas about 'Care', despite all of the research which was based on her theory.

4. The connection to other theories or views
To what degree is a theory based on knowledge from other theories, either within nursing or from other disciplines?

Roy's adaptation-model, for instance, is based on Helson's adaptation-level theory (Roy 1991). Virginia Henderson's classification of fundamental human needs can be found in some nursing theories without any specific reference to Henderson. The influence of the psychologist Maslow can also be detected in these theories.

5. The explicit or implicit assumptions of the theory
These assumptions or presuppositions may be of an ethnic, cultural, social, legal, philosophical or ideological nature, for instance. They may be formulated explicitly by a theorist, but they may also have influenced the theory or the theorist in an implicit way. To be able to use a theory, we need to know what the implications of these presuppositions are in the practical situation. Presuppositions can also be imported from other theories (see point 4).

Van der Bruggen's 'anthropological nursing' (1987) explicitly mentions the philosophical ideas on which the theory is based. The ideas on which 'anthroposophical nursing' is based (van der Bruggen 1992) are also clearly stated. Van den Brink-Tjebbes has based her theory (1989) on Judeo-Christianity and the way it has been interpreted by the philosopher Levinas. Orem's theory (1991) is less explicit in this respect, and while this can give the impression that it is 'philosophically neutral', it is implicitly inspired by the idea (or ideal) of the self-actualizing human being as an individual, autonomous person (see also Grypdonck 1991). This has obvious consequences when using her theory.

6. Views on nursing theories
What are the theorist's views on nursing theories in general and their development, application and testing? Can his own theory contribute to this or live up to his own expectations?

Leininger's views on theories differ in outline from those of her American colleagues; from an epistemological point of view they have more in common with European views like existentialism and phenomenology.

7. What type of theory is it?

A theory's sole aim might be a description of reality, or it's intention may be to explain particular phenomena. It may, in fact, have a number of functions. We need to know the level at which the theory is set (is it, for instance, a situation-producing theory?). We also need to know its scope. Is it set at the more abstract grand-theory level (what part of reality does the theory deal with?).

The theorist's own view of the theory can give some insight here, and we can also look at other authors' comments and form our own impressions. Integrated Nursing is clear about its purpose and level (Koene, Grypdonck and others, 1987). Chapter 3 discusses the different kinds of theories more fully.

8. The four central concepts (meta-paradigms)

Four central concepts (or *meta-paradigms*) are usually distinguished in nursing theories (see section 2.2.5). In evaluating theories, it is important to note how these meta-paradigms are described and how they inter-relate.

This includes such matters as the theoritician's view of how the patient relates to his illness, and what the role of nursing is. When do we describe that activity going on as 'nursing'? When is nursing desirable or necessary? It is also important to know what the author sees as being the *aim* of nursing. We need to understand her or his views on how people relate to their environment, how patient and environment influence each other, and what role the nurse plays in this. The relationship between these factors, and thus the author's views on the central concepts, is presupposed either consciously or subconsciously, and these views can have important implicit and explicit *consequences* in the practical situation. The author may not necessarily be aware of these consequences: for example, the idea of reincarnation, found in many Eastern philosophies, may be taken to mean that death (and sometimes life as well) is an illusion (Maya). This might influence a nurse's attitude to death and dying patients. These four central concepts will not always be discussed as separate elements in a theory, and the reader will often have to trace them through various places in the text.

9. The concepts used in the theory

The specific concepts the theorist uses in a theory are of great importance. It is in this point particularly that theories differ from each other. We need to examine whether the concepts are clearly defined, and how they compare and relate to each other. Can they be easily recognized in the practical situation or are they rather abstract? Often the most important concepts are stated explicitly by the theorist, but sometimes there is a lack of clarity which makes the concepts vague and disputable. The author's views on which are the most important concepts can often be found in the meta-theoretical literature. Not only the concepts which are used count; the way in which they are described and defined is important as well. Anthroposophy, for instance, gives meanings to the words 'mind', 'body' and 'soul' which are very different from the ones they have within a Christian perspective. Conversely, different theories may use different terms to denote nearly identical concepts.

10. Propositions or statements

Further to point nine, we need to describe and analyse the propositions or statements made within the theory. These propositions connect the different concepts, and we need to know whether the propositions are logical and whether they can be tested. To what extent are they based on empirical data or other acceptable principles?

This point seems more straightforward than it really is. There are different types of propositions, and in addition theories at the grand-theory level may contain propositions which cannot possibly be tested by research. It is, however, important to be aware of the statements a theory makes and to examine them as critically as possible.

11. The nursing process

Does the theory describe the nursing process? If so, in what way? If not, can we deduce any views of the nursing process from it? Does the theorist indicate clearly how the nursing process can and should be applied within the practice of direct nursing care? Does the theory give any other concrete indications of how it can be used?

The nursing process is a generally accepted order of nursing conduct, although different authors have used many different kinds of phases when talking about it (see also section 2.2.4).

12. The theory's generality

This is a measure of the extent to which the theory can be generally applied. Is it applicable, for instance, only to certain fields of nursing? Is it aimed at specific care situations, or limited to certain age groups?

Some theories seem to be applicable only within general health care, others are relevant solely or chiefly with certain patients or clients: most theories appear to be mainly aimed at adults. The theorist may clearly indicate this, but where there is no explicit statement the reader must form his own judgment. A theory's generality is not related to its function, level or range. One micro-level theory can have a high degree of generality, independent of the culture in which it is applied, while another (about pain, for instance) may only be applicable within the culture in which it was developed, unless certain cultural differences are taken into account. Similarly, one grand-level theory may be almost universally applicable while another is limited to our Western culture.

13. The theory's usefulness in practice
In assessing the practical usefulness of a theory it is important to be aware of how the theory, or parts of it, has been used within different fields or care situations. This information can be found mainly in the specialist journals, although sometimes when a theory has been around for a while and has been through processes of adjustment, such material may appear in the primary literature. We should be aware, though, of any factors within the practical situation which may determine whether a theory works successfully or not. The success of a theory can be determined, for instance, by the attitude of the people involved in its application.

However, even when a theory has not yet been applied in practice it is possible to form some idea of its potential application. Whether a theory can be successfully applied or not depends partly on the boundaries it identifies, such as the type of theory it is or its degree of generality (see also chapters 5 and 6).

14. Nursing specifics
For insight into the usefulness of a theory, we should also look at what the theory says about certain specific nursing topics, including:

1 Nursing discipline in general;
2 Nursing education;
3 Nursing administration; and
4 Nursing research.

We should investigate whether these subjects are mentioned, and if so how much attention they are given. We can consider the author's opinion about these subjects and note the problems she or he identifies, the developments she or he expects, the kind of change she or he proposes and whether she or he provides any guidelines. (The application of a theory could, for instance, require changes in administration.)

15. The criticism or support the theory has received
It is also useful to investigate any criticism or support the theory has already received, and what arguments or motives have been used

effectively in this process. If necessary, criticism can be classified under the list of headings we are using here. When this is not possible, short comments (with their sources) can be brought together here.

Note that the comments made in section 13 also apply here. Criticism can also be found in the meta-theoretical literature. When the criticism concerns essential parts of the theory this can have a negative effect on its general acceptance and usage. This criticism (but also the level of support it enjoys) should itself be critically investigated in order to find out whether or not it is justified.

This list forms a structured and methodical process by which theories can be evaluated: it can thus be used as an evaluation instrument. Under each heading we can distinguish between a descriptive part and a part which can be used for analysis and criticism. This means that there is a total of thirty questions we can ask. Giving exact answers or fitting a theory into particular categories (deciding, for instance, the level of a theory) is not always possible. Sometimes the theorist will indicate this her or himself and sometimes meta-theorists will have made their judgement known — but opinions may differ. The vital issue is that the reader should learn to make a well-argued choice, which at times may be a provisional one. Students (and other users) should be discouraged from trying to pass definitive judgements about theories. In most cases, there will be endless scope for further fascinating discussion about theories.

Accurate use of the literature is important in evaluation. In the American literature in particular, the most important theorists have been analysed and compared by various authors, each one placing his own emphasis. In the appendices we give an overview of meta-theoretical works and the theories they discuss, and this makes it easier to find the relevant sections. Also in the appendices, you will find a few diagrams from the literature which compare different theories. The aim is to provide a useful aid for the evaluation of theories.

The user of an evaluation instrument such as the one presented here is free to choose which points to develop and which to ignore (it is, after all, only an aid). It is also possible to add new points to the list.

Appendix 6 gives an example of how the evaluation instrument can be used to work on an assignment.

The Vijverberg Evaluation Instrument for Nursing Theories

Comments

The evaluation points discussed in this book have here been put into the form of questions, enabling them to be used as an evaluation instrument. This instrument was initially developed at the Vijverberg-Felua Christian College for Higher Education in Ede by Wil Doornenbal (a psychologist), Peter Blokhuis (a philosopher) and Gert Hunink (a nursing scientist). The user is free to use part or parts of it selectively, in for instance a training assignment or a clinical lesson. The instrument as a whole is fairly extensive. The numbering of the list is intended only as a way of separating the different questions: it is not a strict order in which they should be dealt with. The way and the order in which the questions are used will depend on the theory (or the theorist) under evaluation. A question may be easy to answer when dealing with one theorist yet much more difficult when dealing with another.

The list is divided into two parts. Questions labelled *A* make up the descriptive part, and those labelled *B* deal with analysis and criticism. In the descriptive questions, the idea is to describe or summarise the theoretician's view. Always ask yourself what the theoreticians themselves say about the relevant questions (this means you have to use the primary literature). Look too at what other authors have written about the subject (this involves secondary literature). The latter approach is particularly useful when there appears to be no direct answer in the primary literature.

In the questions aimed at analysis and criticism, try to indicate the stronger and the weaker aspects of the relevant theory, and compare and contrast it with other theories. You will have to refer to the secondary literature, but try to formulate your own ideas as well.

It is important to always be aware whether you are dealing with primary or secondary literature when you are collecting information. Make sure you make correct references to the literature you have consulted. This is important because a concise description or interpretation of a theory in the secondary literature can sometimes give an inaccurate interpretation of the original text.

Purchasers of this book are automatically granted permission to photocopy the following list of questions for their own use, for ease of reference when studying nursing theories.

A Description	*B Analysis and criticism*
A1 How does the theoretician describe his own background and approach, and how is she or he described by other authors? Consider topics such as training and experience (including work-experience) and other factors.	**B1** In what ways have the theorist's experiences, training and background had a positive or negative effect on the theory?
A2 With what aim or purpose in mind was the theory formulated?	**B2** Describe how you feel about the reasons and the aims behind the theory. Does it seem to you that these aims will be met?
A3 Has the theory developed through time, or is it (at the moment) a one-off presentation? If the theory has developed outline the course it has taken, including dates if possible.	**B3** How would you assess the theory's development? Is this development an improvement? If there has been no development so far, in what ways do you think it would be useful or even necessary?
A4 Is there a relationship between this theory and other theories or ideas? To what extent is it based on the knowledge of other authors' work or theories?	**B4** To what extent is the theory based on other theories? Does it use the ideas of other authors without acknowledging them?
A5 On what ideological or philosophical principles and assumptions is the theory explicitly based? What is the nature of these principles and assumptions?	**B5** On what principles or assumptions is the theory implicitly based? What consequences could the principles or assumptions, both implicit and explicit, have? What are their advantages and disadvantages?

A6 What are the theoretician's ideas about scientific nursing theories, about the process of theory development and about the application and testing of theories in general? In what ways does she or he want to contribute to this?

B6 How does the theorist's view agree with or differ from that of other theorists? What are the consequences of this view? Is the theory itself in agreement with the theorist's view? Is it, in its present form, suitable for the aim the theorist has in mind or would a different kind of theory be more suitable?

A7 What type of theory is it with regard to
– the function of the theory,
– the level of the theory, and
– the range of the theory?

B7 Is the theory at a suitable level for its aim? Would it be possible to develop it further, to a higher level? Would it be possible to link the theory to others with a different range? Explain how.

A8 What does the theory say about the following central concepts ('meta-paradigms') and how they interrelate?
a: the human being, person and patient
b: health/illness
c: environment
d: nursing

B8 In what ways do the descriptions of the four central concepts agree with the views of other theorists and how do they differ, both according to the theorist himself and to other authors? Has the relationship between them been clearly and logically described? What are the consequences of defining the concepts in this particular way?

A9 What important concepts is the theory specifically based on? What concrete examples are given?

B9 What are the most important characteristics of the concepts? Have the concepts themselves been clearly defined? How are they distinguished from related or synonymous concepts? Is this description recognizable in the practical situation? Is it used consistently?

A10 How do the most important propositions or statements relate these concepts to each other?

B10 What is the nature of the relationship between the concepts? Are the statements or propositions logical? Have they been well enough argued? Is it possible to test them? To what extent are they based on empirical data?

A11 Is the Nursing Process described? If so, what is said about it? If not, what other guidelines are given about the practical situation? Are there any other specific guides given about the theory's usage?

A12 What does the theory say about its generality; or where and when it can be used? Does it distinguish between the different fields of nursing, or is it thought to be equally useful in all the different fields?

A13 What is known about how the theory (or parts of it) can be applied within the different fields and the levels at which it can be applied (administration, care or research)?

A14 Does the theory say anything about the following?
a: Nursing in general
b: Nursing education
c: Nursing administration
d: Nursing research.

A15 What criticism or support has the theory received? Who has offered this commentary, and what were the arguments and motives used?

B11 What differences and similarities are there between this and the work of other authors with respect to the formulation, content and practice of the Nursing Process? Can it be applied directly within the practical nursing situation?

B12 To which fields or areas of care does the theory principally appear to be applicable? Can it also be used in situations other than those indicated?

B13 What would be your evaluation of the application of this theory? Does the way in which it can be used agree with the intentions of the theory and those of the theoretician her or himself?

B14 To what extent and in what way are nursing, and nursing training, management and research. discussed? What consequences might this have? How does it compare with the work of other theoreticians? Is the theory based on general values as they are formulated in, for instance, the professional codes?

B15 Is the positive or negative criticism of the various parts of the theory unambiguous? Is this criticism related to essential or less essential parts of the theory, or to the theory as a whole? How would you analyse and evaluate the criticism? What are your reasons and arguments for this analysis?

Conclusion

What general conclusions can you make by way of summary? What are the strengths and weaknesses of the theory? Give your own opinion.

Other Evaluation Instruments

To demonstrate other evaluation instruments, we will introduce two of them here: those of the Americans Fawcett and Isenberg.

■ FAWCETT

Fawcett distinguishes between theories and conceptual models and on the basis of this distinction she wrote two separate books. One (1989) is concerned with the analysis and evaluation of conceptual models and the other (1993) with the analysis and evaluation of nursing theories. For various reasons (outlined in appendix 3) we will not use this distinction here: the list below gives Fawcett's 'Framework for analysis and evaluation of conceptual models of nursing'. This instrument has been specifically developed for the analysis of conceptual frameworks, and not for analysis at another level, such as middle-range theories (Fawcett, 1989). She makes a distinction between analysis on the one hand and evaluation on the other, and since her first version in 1980 several alterations have been made to the list.

Questions for analysis
–   What is the historical evolution of the conceptual model?
–   What approach to development of nursing knowledge does the model exemplify?
–   Upon what assumptions was the conceptual model based?
–   How are nursing's meta-paradigm concepts explicated in the model?
  – How is the person defined and described?
  – How is the environment defined and described?
  – How is health defined? How are wellness and illness differentiated?
  – How is nursing defined? What is the goal of nursing? How is the nursing process described?

– What statements are made about the relationships among the four meta-paradigm concepts?
– What areas of concern are identified by the conceptual model?
– What is the source of these concerns?

Questions for evaluation

– Are the assumptions upon which the conceptual model was based made explicit?
– Does the conceptual model provide complete descriptions of all four concepts of nursing's meta-paradigm?
– Do the relational propositions of the conceptual model completely link the four meta-paradigm concepts?
– Is the internal structure of the conceptual model logically congruent?
  – Does the model reflect more than one contrasting world view?
  – Does the model reflect characteristics of more than one category of models?
  – Do the components of the model reflect logical translation of diverse perspectives?
– Does the conceptual model generate empirically testable theories?
– Do tests of derived theories yield evidence in support of the model?
– Is the conceptual model socially congruent?
  – Does the conceptual model, when linked with relevant theories, lead to nursing activities that meet society's expectations or do the expectations created by the conceptual model require societal changes?
– Is the conceptual model socially significant?
  – Does the conceptual model, when linked with relevant theories, lead to nursing actions that make important differences in the person's health status?
– Is the conceptual model socially useful?
  – Does the conceptual model include explicit rules for research, practice, education and administration?
  – Is the conceptual model comprehensive enough to provide direction for research, practice, education and administration when linked with relevant theories?
  – Is the investigator given sufficient direction about what to study and what questions to ask?
  – Is the practitioner able to make pertinent observations, decide that a nursing problem exists, and prescribe and execute a course of action that achieves the goal specified?

– Does the educator have sufficient guidelines to contruct a curriculum, and a reasonable understanding of what knowledge and skills are needed?

– Does the administrator have sufficient guidelines to organize and deliver nursing services?

– What is the overall contribution of the conceptual model to nursing knowledge?

■ ISENBERG

Part 1: analysis of the theory or model on the basis of the following points.

1.1 Determine and describe the most important components ('building blocks').

1.2 Which concepts of the propositions and/or premises are linked, according to the theory?

1.3 The 'paradigm of Nursing Science' consist (according to many authors) of four 'essential concepts': person, environment, health and illness, and nursing.

a: How have these four concepts been defined?

b: How has the relation between person and environment been described?

c: Is there a clear distinction between health and illness?

1.4 What are the theoretician's views concerning nursing as a profession, a discipline, and a science?

Part 2; evaluation of the theory or the model on the basis of the following points.

2.1 The logical consistency:

a: reflect on the choice for either a matrix or a model;

b: label the concepts and formalize the premises and propositions;

c: accommodate the formalized concepts in a matrix or model;

d: determine whether there are any contradictory or unmentioned relations;

e: determine the character of the relations.

2.2 The extent to which it can can be tested:

a: to what extent are the concepts operationalized?

b: to what extent have testable hypotheses been derived from the theory?

c: what is the theory's scope? Explain.

d: what is the theory's generality? Explain.

Part 3: the theory's usefulness:

3.1   The usefulness for the practical situation of nursing care.
   a: What is, within this theory, the aim of nursing?
   b: How has the nursing process been described?
   c: When using this theory in the practical situation:
       – what categories of patient-data are included in the nursing dossier?
       – what is the character of the nursing diagnosis?
       – what is the character of the nursing care?
       – what is the character of the evaluation of the nursing care?
3.2   The usefulness for the practise of nursing scientific research:
   a: What is the aim/task of the nursing research within this theory?
   b: How is the research-process described?

A Clarification of Concepts

Science in general has its own jargon, and so does nursing science. Those interested in reading more about the subject will soon discover that concepts are not always used unambiguously, and definitions vary. This is largely to be expected: the definition of a word such as 'science' is determined by a number of assumptions. Therefore, to set some guidelines to the meaning of concepts such as 'theory' and 'model', we will briefly discuss a few concepts here (we have used an appendix for this purpose to avoid interruption of the flow of the text). We do not aim to give any absolute definition of the concepts, but rather to offer some insight into the different ways in which they are used. Their interpretation can be based on mutual agreement, personal preferences or both, as well as on the underlying epistemological ideas. The broad descriptions and different views given here should encourage questioning of the context and of the author's meaning each time a concept is used. For an extensive discussion of the various concepts, refer to Powers and Knapp (1990).

Science
There are many definitions and views of 'science' in circulation, influenced by various underlying assumptions, and we cannot discuss them all. One practical and fairly common definition is that *science is the whole of the activities aimed at the acquisition of scientific knowledge.*

Scientific knowledge is of a special character, and not all knowledge can be thus described. It is not primary: it presupposes non-scientific knowledge. The transition from non-scientific to scientific knowledge is a fluid one. This can be illustrated by the development of science. It is impossible to say when exactly a branch of science becomes a 'real science'. Broadly speaking, the *tools* of science are research and the development of theories. Scientific training is important for the transmission of scientific views and knowledge about research and theory development, and to train scientists in the methods of acquiring knowledge in a particular field. Amongst the characteristics of scientific method we often find a systematic approach, reasoning, a public nature and an aim for objectivity. Many books have been published about 'science' as a subject, and there is even a 'science of science': epistemology deals with the philosophy, sociology and history of science.

Nursing science

Nursing science can be described as 'that branch of science which is concerned with nursing', that is, the branch of science concerned with the study of nursing or the domain of knowledge related to nursing practice. According to Huijer Abu-Saad (1990) this domain of nursing is mainly concerned with the following:

1 the recognition and analysis of real or potential health problems;
2 the definition of some health problems as nursing problems;
3 therapeutic interventions which aim to alleviate or prevent these problems;
4 study and analysis of environmental factors which influence the promotion and maintenance of health.

Some would define nursing science as the caring science. 'Care', in all its aspects and forms (including non-professional care) is the central subject of study. This offers an interesting perspective and extends the domain and relevance of nursing science.

Nursing science is a 'practical science'. As far as its content and method is concerned, however, it is related to the so-called social sciences (like sociology and psychology) rather than the natural sciences (like physics and biology). Medical science, on the other hand, is strongly related to, and influenced by, the natural sciences.

Paradigm

'Paradigm' is an important concept used by Thomas Kuhn (an American physicist) in 1970, and adopted by many others. Kuhn formulated an influential theory dealing with the development of science in which the concept 'paradigm' has an important place. He used the term in various meanings, including:

 – a characteristic example, or *exemplar*;
 – the epistemological views of a particular school;
 – a research programme;

- the specific research methods of a science;
- as a synonym of theory.

Even within nursing, the meaning of this concept is ambiguous. When we speak of the nursing paradigms or meta-paradigms, we usually mean the four concepts which are thought to be central to nursing (see section 2.2).

Incommensurable paradigms are those which are incompatible within a scientific area or between different scientific areas, and their presence makes meaningful discussion almost impossible because they can hardly be compared, being of a different order. According to Kuhn, the discipline is in a pre-paradigmatic (or *not yet scientific*) phase at that moment. This idea has almost become a dogma. Our observations cannot be objective because they are coloured by a specific paradigm, and a different paradigm will reveal other factors or interpret the same factors in a different way (see also section 4.2).

Theory
The word 'practice' is derived from the Greek for *to do*; 'theory' is derived from *theorio*: to consider, assess, or think through ('theatre' is derived from the same root). The usage of this word is rather diverse, and depends on the context in which it is used. We want to use the concept in its more or less scientific meaning, rather than its vague definition of 'knowledge from books', or 'instructions for practice' (see also section 2.1). In short, *theory* deals with the statements made about part or the whole of reality. More precisely, it is a systematic set of statements concerning a phenomenon or a number of phenomena in a certain field.

A theory consists of one or more concepts, related together by propositions (the concepts can be thought of as the building blocks of the theory, and the statements as the mortar which holds them together). For convenience, we will use this general description of 'theory' (and also of 'view' and 'model') here.

There is also dispute about when exactly a theory can be labelled 'scientific'. According to a certain school of thought within the philosophy of science, this can only occur once it has been tested through research. Others believe that this kind of approach is inappropriate for the social sciences. At the grand-theory level the theory is too broad and abstract to be researched as a whole. It is possible to research parts of it, but this does not test the theory as a whole.

It can do little harm, though, to research the main points of a theory: when parts of it can be supported by research it may improve its chances of

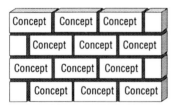

Figure A1 *Concepts can be regarded as the building blocks of a theory. The statements link the concepts and can be regarded as the mortar.*

acceptance. In this respect, the kind of theory in question is also relevant. A prescriptive theory, for instance, cannot be researched through descriptive investigation of the current practical situation. (There is much more to say about this, but it is outwith the scope of this book.)

Model

In nursing theorizing, we often speak of a *model* rather than a *theory*. The discussion surrounding the definitions of these concepts tends to be chaotic and confusing. A *conceptual model* (or *framework*) is, according to several authors, comparable to a 'grand-theory'. The term 'model' is used in a variety of ways. Often it is used to signify a broad abstraction which does not include all the available factors, and it is then a simplification or a reduction of reality rather than a comprehensive representation of it. It is thus generally thought that a model cannot be tested as fully as a theory. The word is also used when a new theory is beginning to emerge. Usually, however, the only difference between theory and model is linguisitic, and of no practical significance at all. Note, though, that Fawcett especially maintains a sharp distinction between a theory and a model.

However, the word 'model' is also used to mean a symbolic, schematic or graphic reproduction of some aspect of reality. Examples of this include pictograms, organizational charts (see figure A2) and anatomical models. A theory can contain one or more of this type of model. Leininger's 'Sunrise Model' is a model which schematically reproduces the main principles of her theory.

Concept

Concept is a term or a label used to describe a phenomenon or a group of phenomena. It may refer to matters which can be observed directly as well as those which cannot. 'Happiness' and 'intelligence' cannot be observed directly yet few will doubt their existence. A concept like 'chair', on the other hand, refers to objects which can be observed directly. A concept can be specific or general: the concept of a *dining-room chair* is more specific than that of a *chair*, and the concept of *furniture* is more

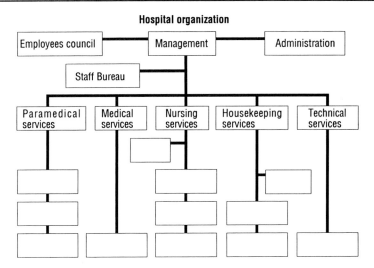

Figure A2 *An organizational chart is an example of a schematic model. It is a way of depicting some aspect of reality.*

general still. Concepts can be described in various ways, and scientific usage or professional jargon in particular differ from every day usage.

Certain concepts can also vary widely across the different professions. For example, the concept of *depression* is entirely different in cardiology, psychiatry and meteorology. Concepts can be regarded as the building blocks from which theories are built up. Scientific concepts have to be defined more precisely so that we can test them. Definitions are often based on mutual agreement. Even within a specific discipline, concepts might have different meanings. Orem's definition of self-care, for instance, differs from the definition given by the NANDA. Concepts should always, therefore, be considered within a particular context. For the sake of clarity, we should add that the term 'concept' is *not* used in the sense of a provisional plan or idea.

Construct
The term 'construct' is also used regularly, usually to refer to concepts which have been invented or constructed. This means we are dealing with a new concept. Within theorizing there can be times when it is necessary to devise a new term because the ones which already exist are confusing. The concept of 'self-care agency' (Orem) and 'cognator-and-regulator subsystems' (Roy) are examples of constructs.

A Bibliography
of Theorists

This bibliography contains most of the English writing theorists who have produced nursing theories (see also table 1 of appendix 5) and several Dutch nursing theories. Some references are to the original and only publication, but in a number of cases publication was preceded by the appearance in specialist journals of articles dealing with elements from the theory. These articles have not been taken into account here, but the theorists themselves refer to them in the primary literature. In other cases we mention the most recently revised edition (Orem's theory, for instance, is currently in its fourth revision). The bibliography is not comprehensive, and naturally it only gives a picture of the moment when it was compiled. In meta-theoretical literature there are extensive references to other relevant books and articles, and as one reference leads to another a large amount of literature can be discovered. To prevent a lot of searching, it is a good idea to establish a databank of articles from specialist journals. When, for instance, Roy's adaptation theory is used within an institution, all the known literature about it can be kept in a central, accessible place. It is also important that the literature is used correctly and full references to the sources are given.

Bergen B van, Hollands L *Naar een profiel van der verpleegkundige* Lochem: De Tijdstroom (1975)

Brink-Tjebbes J A van den *Verpleging naar de maat – een verplegingswetenschappelijke optiek* Lochem: De Tijdstroom (1989) (includes a summary in English: *Nursing in respect of the higher rules pertaining to nursing*)

Bruggen H van der *Naar een antropologische verpleegkunde* Lochem: De Tijdstroom (1976)

Henderson V *Textbook of the principles and practice of nursing. The nature of nursing.* New York: Macmillan (1978)

Johnson DE *The behavioural system model for nursing* in Riehl JP, Roy C (eds) *Conceptual Models for Nursing Practice* 2nd edition, New York: Appleton-Century-Crofts (1980)

King I *A theory for nursing: systems, concepts, process* New York: Wiley (1981)

Koene G, Grypdonck M, Rodenbach M Th, Windey T *Integrerende Verpleegkunde: Wetenschap in de Praktijk* Lochem: De Tijdstroom (1989). For an English article on this theory see Grypdonck M, Koene G, Rodenbach M Th, Windey T and Blaupain JE *Integrating nursing: a holistic approach to the delivery of nursing care* International Journal of Nursing Studies, 16, 1979, 215–230

Leininger M *Transcultural nursing concepts, theories and practices* New Jersey: Slack (1978)

Leininger M (ed) *Culture care diversity & universality: a theory of nursing* New York: National League for Nursing (1991)

Levine ME *Introduction to clinical nursing* Philadelphia: Davis (1973)

Neuman B *The Neuman systems model* Norwalk: Appleton & Lange (1989)

Newman MA *Theory development in nursing* Philadelphia: Davis (1979)

Nightingale F *Notes on nursing: what it is and what it is not* (1859, republished in various editions and collections)

Orem DE *Nursing: concepts of practice* St Louis: Mosby (1991)

Orlando IJ *The dynamic nurse-patient relationship* New York: Putnam's Sons (1972)

Parse RR *Man–living–health: a theory of nursing* New York: Wiley (1981)

Paterson JG, Zderad LT *Humanistic nursing* New York: National League for Nursing (1988)

Peplau HE *Interpersonal relations in nursing* New York: Putnam's Sons (1952)

Riehl JP *The Riehl interaction model* in Riehl, Sisca (eds) *Conceptual models for nursing practice* 3rd edition, New York: Appleton-Century-Crofts (1989)

Rogers ME *An introduction to the theoretical basis of nursing* Philadelphia: Davis (1970)

Roy C *The Roy adaptation model; the definitive statement* Norwalk: Appleton & Lange (1991)

Travelbee J *Interpersonal aspects of nursing* Philadelphia: Davis (1971)

Watson J *Nursing: the philosophy and science of caring* Boston: Little Brown (1979)

Watson J *Nursing: human science and human care* East Norwalk: Appleton-Century-Crofts (1985)

Wiedenbach E *Clinical nursing: a helping art* New York: Springer-Verlag (1964)

Tables

The following informative tables have either been taken from the litera-ture directly, or have been based on it. Most tables are random pictures; none claim to be exhaustive. They aim to help the reader who is collecting further information about the different theories.

Table A1 *Nursing theorists writing in English, their most important publications and the date when they appeared (in some cases including articles which outline the basic principles of a theory). Dates of later publications which elaborate on the same theory are also given. The table is not exhaustive: for complete book references see appendix 4. (Based on Meleis 1991, Walker & Avant 1988 and Marriner-Tomey 1989.)*

Theorist	Year	Title	Later publications
Florence Nightingale †	1859	Notes on Nursing: What it is and what it is not	
Hildegarde Peplau	1952	Interpersonal relations in nursing	1962, 1963, 1969
Virginia Henderson	1955	Textbook of the principles and practice of nursing *(with B Harmer)*	
	1966	The nature of nursing	1972, 1978
Dorothea Johnson	1959	A philosophy of nursing	1961, 1966, 1974
	1980	The behavioural system model for nursing	
Faye Abdellah	1960	Patient-centred approaches to nursing	1965,1973
Ida Jean Orlando	1961	The dynamic nurse-patient relationship	

Theorist	Year	Title	Later publications
Ernestine Wiedenbach	1964	Clinical nursing: a helping art	1967, 1969, 1970, 1977
Joyce Travelbee †	1964	Interpersonal aspects of nursing	1969, 1971, 1979
	1969	Interventions in psychiatric nursing	
Myra Levine	1966	Adaptation and assessment	1969, 71, 73
	1967	Introduction to clinical nursing	
Imogene King	1968	A conceptual framework of reference for nursing	1975
	1971	Toward a theory for nursing: general concepts of human behaviour	
	1981	A theory for nursing: systems, concepts, process	
Martha Rogers †	1970	An introduction to the theoretical basis of nursing	1980
Sister Callista Roy	1970	Adaptation: a conceptual framework for nursing	1974, 1976, 1980, 1984
	1991	The Roy adaptation model: the definitive statement	
Madeleine Leininger	1970	Nursing and anthropology: two worlds to blend	1980, 1981, 1984, 1985
	1978	Transcultural nursing: concepts, theories and practices	
	1991	Cultural care diversity and universality: a theory of nursing	
Dorothea Orem	1971	Nursing: concepts of practice	1981, 1982, 1985, 1991
Betty Neuman	1972	The Betty Neuman healthcare systems model	1989
Josephine Patterson & Loretta Zderad	1976	Humanistic nursing	1988
Margaret Newman	1979	Toward a theory of health	
	1986	Health as expanding consciousness	
Rosemary Parse	1981	Man–living–health: a theory for nursing	
Jean Watson	1985	Nursing: human science and human care	

† Now deceased

Table A2 *Nursing theorists writing in English who inspired European nurses, based upon a brief review of the European nursing literature (according to van der Bruggen, 1992).*

Theorist	Belgium	Denmark	Finland	France	Great Britain	(former) Yugoslavia	The Netherlands	Norway	Portugal	Spain	Sweden	Switzerland
Henderson	■	■	■	■	■	■	■	■	■	■	■	■
King		■	■				■					
Leininger					■		■					
Newman		■	■		■							
Nightingale			■									
Orem	■	■	■	■	■		■	■	■	■	■	■
Orlando		■	■				■					
Peplau		■	■							■		
Roy		■	■	■	■		■			■	■	■
Rogers	■	■	■							■		
Roper			■	■	■							■
Travelbee		■										■
Watson					■							

Table A3 *An overview of discussions (or references) in English of several leading nursing theories in meta-theoretical literature.*

Theoretician	Barnum (1994)	Chinn & Kramer (1991)	Fawcett (1989)	Fawcett (1993)	Marriner-Tomey (1989)	Meleis (1991)	Nicoll (1992)	Parse (1987)	Pepper & Leddy (1993)	Riehl Sisca (1989)	Walker & Avant (1988)	Walsh (1991)	Wesley (1992)
Henderson		3			■	12	7				1	1	■
Johnson	16	1	■	2	■	■	23		■		2		■
King	15	3	■	2	■	■	10	■	■	■	2	■	■
Leininger	8	1		■	■	3	7		■	1	1		■
Levine	15	4	■	2	■	■	2			■	1		■
Neuman	5	2	■	2	■	■	3	2	■	■	2	2	■
Newman	21	3		■	■	16	9	1	■		2		1
Nightingale	1	3			■	10	6	1	1	8			■
Orem	11	3	■	2	■	■	9	■	■	■	1	■	■
Orlando	7	2		■	■	■	6			6	2	1	■
Parse	5	1		■	■		3	■	■	2			■
Paterson & Zderad	5	2			■	4/5	1		1				■
Peplau	4	2		■	■	10	5		■		1	1	■
Riehl-Sisca					■	4	7			■	2		1
Rogers	17	2	■	2	■	■	23	■	■	■	3		■
Roper												■	
Roy	20	3	■	2	■	■	14	■	■	■	7	■	■
Travelbee		3			■	■					1		1
Watson	22	2		■	■		10		■	■	2		■
Wiedenbach	2	2			■	■	17				2		■

See foot of facing page for key

Table A4 *Some authors and editors who have done work on nursing theories at meta-theoretical level. The year given is that of the latest edition, which may be a revision (for complete references see the bibliography).*

Author(s)	Year	Title
Barnum BJ	1994	Nursing theory analyses, application, evaluation
Chinn PC & Kramer MK	1991	Theory and nursing: a systematic approach
Fawcett J	1989	Analysis and evaluation of conceptual models of nursing
Fawcett J	1993	Analysis and evaluation of nursing theories
Leddy S & Pepper MJ	1993	Conceptual bases of professional nursing
Marriner-Tomey A	1989	Nursing theorists and their work
Meleis AI	1991	Theoretical nursing: development and progress
Nicoll LA (ed)	1992	Perspectives on nursing theory
Parse RR	1987	Nursing science: major paradigms, theories and critiques
Riehl-Sisca J (formerly Riehl) & Roy	1989	Conceptual models for nursing practice
Walker LO & Avant KC	1988	Strategies for theory construction in nursing
Walsh M	1991	Models in clinical nursing – the way forward
Wesley RL	1992	Nursing theories and models

A few of these authors have also been involved in formulating their *own* theory. The list is incomplete, but much literature can also be found in the various nursing journals. The authors mentioned above regularly refer to these articles in their books. In particular Meleis gives an extensive bibliography and summaries of a few important articles. Nicoll has integrated a large number of articles from the 1950s which are related to, and have influenced, nursing science in his book. Each article is followed by a commentary by the relevant author(s) about their views at the time of publication. Thus, the book shows an interesting development in views on nursing in the US over the past few decades. Walker and Avant do not concentrate on one or a few theories. As they too regularly refer to the various theories, they have been included in this list (this applies to Barnum and Chinn & Kramer as well).

Key to table A3
■ indicates discussion of the theory
Figures indicate references to the theory or the theorist (sometimes including references to other works of the theorist)
See also appendix 4 and table 4 of appendix 5.
Some of the meta-theorists discuss several other theories besides the ones mentioned here.

The following tables (A5 to A9) contain classifications of theories by various authors. The classification of theory types in chapter 3 is mainly based on the form, rather than the content, of the theories. These tables classify theories according to content. They are not, however, absolute: differences of opinion about whether a theory should be included in one category or another are possible.

Table A5 *Classification of nursing theories on the basis of the emphasis that is put on one or more essential concepts (based on Newman).*

Emphasis on environment	Nightingale (1859),
Emphasis on the interaction between client and nursing	Peplau (1952), Orlando (1961), King (1971)
Emphasis on the client	Henderson (1966), Orem (1971), Johnson (1961), Roy (1971)
Emphasis on the client and the environment	Rogers (1970)
Emphasis on health	Beckstrand (1978), Smith (1979), Newman (1979)

Table A6 *Classification based on paradigmatic origin.*

	Development models	System models	Interaction models
1984	Peplau Orlando	Johnson Roy Rogers King Neuman	Riehl
1989	Rogers Watson Parse	Roy King Neuman	Riehl Levine Orem

The *development models* are based on the theories of Erikson, Freud, Maslow, Peplau, Carl Rogers, Sullivan and the behaviourist school (Bijou and Baer). *System models* are based on system-theoretical principles. The *interaction models* are related to the symbolic-interaction theory. It is not clear to us from the references whether the original classification is by Johnson (1974) quoted by Meleis (1991), or by Riehl and Roy (1974). In the table the classifications used by Riehl and Roy in 1984, and later by Riehl in 1989, have been combined. For a further explanation of the different categories, see Riehl (1989).

Table A7 *Classification of theories according to the different schools of thought in the period 1950 to 1970 (based on Meleis).*

Needs theorists	Interaction theorists	Outcome theorists
Abdellah	King	Johnson
Henderson	Orlando	Levine
Orem	Paterson & Zderad	Rogers
	Peplau	Roy
	Travelbee	
	Wiedenbach	

This classification is according to Meleis. The theoreticians in the first column concentrate mainly on the needs of those seeking care and try to answer the question 'What do nurses do?' They are not directly medically orientated, but have based their theories on Maslow's heirarchy of needs and are influenced by Erickson's stages of development. These theoreticians all studied at the University of Columbia. The second column lists those who sought to answer the question '*How* do nurses do what they do?' Peplau was the first one to address this question. She sought to link her theory with psychoanalytical theory, and remained closer to the bio-medical model. Development was regarded as an interactive process which focused on the development of the relationship between patient and nurse. The theories were based on interactionism, phenomenology and existentialism. Those in the third column were mainly concerned with the *why* of nursing care. They concentrated on the outcome of the nursing care and the perception of the recipient of the care. The aim of the care was to restore a balance, stability and preservation of energy, or to promote harmony between an individual and his environment. The models are based on system, adaptation and development theories. Nursing is regarded as having the function of an external regulating mechanism (Meleis, 1991).

Table A8 *Classification according to the primary focus of the theories (based on Melleis 1991).*

Nursing clients	Human being/ environment interactions	Interactions	Nursing therapeutics
Johnson	Rogers	King	Levine
Roy		Orlando	Orem
Neuman		Patterson & Zderad	
		Travelbee	
		Wiedenbach	

The theories which have the client (or patient) as their primary focus offer an extensive analysis of the client from a nursing perspective. Rogers mainly concentrates on the relationship between clients and their environment. The third category has as its primary focus the characteristics, elements and types of interaction between clients and nurses. The fourth category focuses on interventions by nurses: the nurse's conduct and the conditions it should meet. These theories offer a framework for interventions (Meleis 1991).

Table A9 *Classification according to central themes (based on Marriner-Tomey 1989).*

The evolution of nursing theory development

Art and Science of	Nightingale	1860s
Humanistic Nursing	Abdellah	1960s– 70s
	Wiedenbach	1960s
	Hall	1960s
	Henderson	1960s
	Leininger	1970s – 80s
	Orem	1970s – 80s
	Adam	1980s
	Watson	1979 –80s
	Parse	1980s
	Benner	1980s
Interpersonal	Peplau	1950s
relationships	Orlando	1960s
	Travelbee	1970s
	Barnard	1970s – 80s
	Mercer	1970s – 80s
	Riehl	1980s
	Erickson, Tomlin & Swain	1980s
Energy	Levine	1960s – 70s
fields	Fitzpatrick	1970s – 80s
	Rogers	1970s – 80s
	Newman	1979 – 80s
Systems	Roy	1970s – 80s
	King	1970s – 80s
	Neuman	1970s – 80s
	Johnson	1980s

Marriner's classification has some overlaps with those of tables A4 – A6. She regards the classification as a chronological one, an evolution of nursing theories: first came a nursing philosophy (Nightingale), then an emphasis on interpersonal relationships (Peplau, Orlando, Travelbee, Mercer), then the art and science of nursing (Henderson, Wiedenbach, Hall), after which scientific aspects of nursing are emphasised for the first time (Abdellah). These were followed by a systems approach which emphasised scientific factors (Johnson, Neuman, Roger, King, Orem, Roy, Barnard) and the philosophy of humanistic nursing which again became important (Watson, Leininger, Parse, Benner). Marriner gives only a summary justification for the classification, but she does give examples using various theories. In her chapter division she classifies Wiedenbach in the second category, while in her general text and the above table she places her in the first category. She does state, however, that the categories are not mutually exclusive. Marriner's scientific and philosophical approach appears to be neo-positivistic. She advocates the reconciliation and extensive testing of theories in order to look for the truth.

Assignment

We have included this assignment to show how the Vijverberg Evaluation Instrument (the ENT) can be used in a concrete way in education. (It is preferable to use this assignment after one or more periods of work placement.) This is followed by an account of our experiences in using the assignment (which might also be useful to practising nurses).

Comments on the assignment
In this book, the word 'theory' is used in a broad sense. It is worth considering the views of some authors who have not necessarily aimed at the formulation of a scientific theory. Before starting on this assignment, the first seven chapters of the book should have been studied, and discussed if possible (ensure that you are also familiar with the comments on the evaluation instrument.)

Aims
The assignment should help achieve the following.
1 Using an evaluation instrument will help the student develop the skill of examining nursing theories systematically. The student gains an opportunity to apply meta-theoretical knowledge.
2 Applying the instrument to a specific theory will develop the student's knowledge of and insight into this theory.
3 By discussing theories with others, the student will acquire knowledge about other theories and will form a view about the theories presently in use.
4 The student will learn to look critically at both theory and practice, and to think about the principles, aims and practice of the profession. He will also learn to form opinions and discuss them with other students or colleagues.
5 The assignment will help the student prepare for his final project.

The skills and knowledge acquired can be applied in practice in the future, and the student will learn to develop individual views about the working of a particular unit and identify a suitable organization model, theory, and policy.

Procedure

The students should divide the theories amongst themselves. In groups of two or three, they should answer both parts (A and B) of the following questions with respect to the particular theory they are working on.

1, 2, (3), 4, 5, 7, 8, 9, 10, 11, 12, (13), 15

For the questions in brackets, answers are usually easy to find but they are not compulsory for the assignment. Answers should be kept brief. It is usually best when the A and B parts are dealt with together, rather than all the As first and then all the Bs. Finally, general conclusion should be given, and the students should add any remarks they want to make. Answers should be typed on a maximum of six A4 pages (not including the bibliography and any possible illustrations). These answers should be photocopied and distributed to the other students and the tutor during the lesson preceding the presentation (or, in the case of a clinical lesson, handed out to the other members of the team). Students should study each other's answers, write down any questions or comments, and compare and contrast the other theories with the one they have studied themselves.

Literature

Use the literature you have, and try to find other relevant literature in the library (see the bibliographies in the appendices, especially table 3 from appendix 5). On the basis of these lists, you can search for further literature. Information can also be found in the various nursing journals. Concentrate on using primary literature (that written by the theoretician himself) and when you use secondary literature be aware that the account of the theory might be coloured by the author's interpretation (and that this might be wrong). You should always add a bibliography when evaluating theories, so that you can always retrace a passage afterwards, and so that others will have the opportunity to refer to the sources you have used. (The articles by Aggleton & Chalmers (1986), for instance, contain some incorrect interpretations, and it is important to know whether they have contributed to the conclusions drawn.)

Presentation

The presentation itself will not be assessed or marked. We would advise the use of a blackboard or OHP. The presentation should take around twenty minutes, of which at least five minutes should be set aside for discussion. The tutor may wish to emphasize particularly important aspects or introduce any interesting aspects which have been omitted.

Assessment
The written part of the assignment may be used as the final project for the nursing theories part of the course.

Experiences
In this section we will discuss the experiences we have had with this material and with the Vijverberg ENT since it was first published, using it with two groups of part-time students and eight groups of full-time students. Firstly, we should examine how can it be used within the existing curriculum of professional training. During the first year, our students are introduced to the areas of views and theories. Subsequently, during the third year both full-time and part-time students carry out the above assignment using the evaluation instrument for theorizing and research. In total, the subject was allocated 100 hours (now increased to 120), of which about 20 lessons are used for theorizing and approximately 40 hours are allocated to self-study. By then, the students will have done two work placements and be able to look back critically at their practical experience.

The Vijverberg ENT is too elaborate for students to be able to work through it in its entirety. They can choose from a number of theories and, in groups of two or three, investigate their chosen theory on the basis of the evaluation instrument. The appendices offer the students a guide to the information available, and use of the library is obviously an indispensable part of the work. It has now been equipped satisfactorily and contains most of the primary and relevant secondary literature and several specialist journals. The students distribute written accounts of their responses to the evaluation points amongst each other, and these written accounts form part of their assessments. They also have to give a presentation of their findings, followed by discussion of the theory which they were investigating. Thus, they learn to identify differences and similarities, and have the opportunity to explore a specific theory in depth but also become acquainted with others. In this way the problem of whether to study one theory in depth or several theories superficially is overcome.

These are not our only aims. The evaluation instrument, in particular, gives an opportunity to develop the skill of looking and thinking critically about nursing. It also encourages students to form their own opinions.

Amongst other things they learn to consult and refer to both the primary and secondary literature. This lays the basis for their final projects and allows them to develop their own opinions about their future profession.

Another important aim of evaluation in nursing training is the teaching of a skill which will, in the future, enable students to explore theories and apply them in practice. They learn to look at and think about theories and their practical consequences in a systematic and structured way, and with this ability they can contribute to discussions about the practical use of theories or theoretical views within an institution. They might, for instance, respond by organizing clinical lessons or starting a study group.

When a particular theory is to be introduced, they will be able to deal with it in a critical manner. This may make it possible to avoid limiting the introduction of a theory to a number of organizational principles, while the institutions and carers think it has been fully implemented. Training in this way fulfils a very real function in promoting the adequate application of nursing theories to the practical field, and we hope it will encourage justice to be done to the theoretician's intentions. Students can also be offered the opportunity to study a single theory using the evaluation instrument as part of a final project. The student can then emphasize how the theory can be applied in practice. Students can also interview nurses who work with a specific theory to gain an insight into their opinions and views.

During our evaluations of the assignments it appeared that students see their work with the ENT as a positive experience (though, as usual, lack of time was sometimes commented on as a negative factor). On the main, students are well motivated to work on the assignments, the written part is usually satisfactory and the presentations tend to be clear and original, though the quality of the discussion tends to vary. It does make a significant difference when the tutor concerned has a thorough knowledge of the theory under discussion.

Bibliography

Barnum B *Nursing theory – analyses, application, evaluation* fourth edition. Philadelphia: Lippincott (1994)

Beukel A van den *De dingen hebben hun geheim, gedachten over natuurkunde, mens en God* Barn: Ten Have (1990)

Bruggen H van der (ed) *De delta van den Nederlandse verpleging* third edition. Lochem: Tijdstroom (1992)

Chinn PL & Kramer MK *Theory and nursing: a systematic approach* St Louis: Mosby (1991)

Christensen PJ & Kenney JW *The nursing process – application of conceptual models* third edition. London: Mosby (1990)

Dickoff J & James P *A theory of theories: a position paper* Nursing Research, 17, 197–203 (1968)

Dickoff J, James P & Wiedenbach *Theory in a practice discipline part 1: practice oriented theory* Nursing Research, 17, 415–35 (1968)

Evers GCM *Theorieën en principes van verpleegkunde – inleiding voor het wetenschappelijk onderwijs en onderzoek* Assen: Van Goercum ((1991)

Fawcett J & Downs FS *The relationship of theory and research* Norwalk: Appleton-Century-Crofts (1968)

Fawcett J *Analyses and evaluation of conceptual models of nursing* Philadelphia: FA Davis (1989)

Fawcett J *Analyses and evaluation of nursing theories* Philadelphia: FA Davis (1993)

Gennep ATG van (ed) *Inleiding tot de orthopedagogiek – facetten van hulpverlening bi opvoedingsproblemen* Meppel: Boom (1988)

Gordon M *Nursing diagnosis: process and application* New York: McGraw Hill (1987)

Grypdonck M *De betekenis van het theoretische pluralisme voor de verpleegkunde* Gezondheid an samenleving, 1, 2–10 (1981)

Grypdonck M *Verpleegkunde theorieën kiezen vanuit christelijk perspectief?* in Mey J de (ed) *Het verpleegkundig beroep in beeld – mensbeelden in de verpleegkunde* Zwolle: Gereformeerde Hogeschool (1991)

Huijer Abu-Saad H *Verplegingswetenschap en de verpleegkundige praktijk; een onderlinge relatie* Verpleegkunde, 4, 181–90 (1990)

Hunink GH & Meijer M (eds) *Symposium verplegingswetenschap –verplegingswetenschap in relatie tot management, praktijk en onderwijs* Leiden: Spruyt, Van Mantgem & De Does (1992)

Hunink GH *Een evaluatie-instrument voor verpleegkundige theorieën – een gids voor het oerwoud* Verpleegkundig Onderwijs, (3), 56–66 (1994)

International Council of Nurses *Nursing next advance: an international classification for nursing practice (ICNP): a working paper* Geneva: ICN (1993)

Iowa Intervention Project, McCloskey JC, Bulecheck GM (eds) *Nursing interventions classification (NIC)* St Louis: Mosby

Iowa Intervention Project *Taxonomy of nursing interventions* Iowa: University of Iowa

Iowa Intervention Project *NIC interventions linked to NANDA nursing diagnosis* Iowa: University of Iowa

Jaarsma T, Dassen T *The relaionship of nursing theory and research: the state of the art* Journal of Advanced Nursing, 18, 783–7 (1993)

Kitson AK (ed) *Nursing art and science* London: Chapman & Hall (1993)

Kuypers WB *Hoe verpleegkundigen genezen – met het hart op de tong* Baarn: Nelissen (1988)

Latour B *Science in Action* Milton Keynes: Open University Press (1987)

Leddy S, en Pepper MJ *Conceptual bases of professional nursing* third edition. Philadelphia: Lippincott (1993)

Linneman E *Wissenschaft oder meinung* Hansler Verlag (1985)

Madsen KB *De ontwikkeling van de psychologie –van speculatieve filosofie tot experimentele wetenschap* Rotterdam: Kooyker (1975)

Meleis AI *Theoretical nursing – development & progress* Philadelphia: Lippincott (1991)

Marr H, Giebing H *Quality assurance in nursing – concepts, methods and case studies* Edinburgh: Campion Press (1994)

Marriner-Tomey A *Nursing theorists and their work* St Louis: Mosby (1989)

National League for Nursing *Theory developemnt: what, why and how* New York: National League for Nursing (1978)

Nicoll LH (ed) *Perspectives on nursing theory* second edition. New York: Lippincott

North American Nursing Diagnosis Association *Taxonomy I revised* St Louis: NANDA (1990)

Ouweneel WJ *Psychologie – een christelijke kijk op het mentale leven* Amsterdam: Buijten & Schipperheijn (1984)

Parse RR *Nursing science – major paradigms, theories and critiques* Philadelphia: WB Saunders (1987)

Powers BA, Knapp TR *A dictionary of nursing theory and research* Newbury Park: Sage (1990)

Reuling A *Methodologieën – een inleiding in onderzoeksstrategieën* Baarn: Nelissen (1986)

Riehl JP, Roy C (eds) *Conceptual models for nursing practice* New York: Appleton & Lange (1989)

Rodgers & Knafl *Concept development in nursing* London: Saunders (1993)

Stouw G (ed) *Holisme: alles of niets?* Kampen: Kok (1990)

Strien PJ van *Praktijk als wetenschap, methodologie van het sociaal – wetenschappelijk handelen* (1985)

Torres G *Theoretical foundations of nursing* Norwalk: Appleton-Century-Crofts (1986)

Veling K *Verpleegkundigen kijken verder. Een christelijk visie op verplegeing* in Mey J de (ed) *Het verpleegkundig beroep in beeld – mensbeelden in de verpleegkunde* Zwolle: Gereformeerde Hogeschool (1991)

Walker LO, Avant KC *Strategies for theory construction in nursing* Norwalk: Appleton & Lange (1988)

Walsh M *Models in clinical nursing – the way forward* London: Saunders (1991)

Walsh M, Ford P *Nursing rituals: research and rational actions* Oxford: Butterworth-Heinemann (1990)

Wesley RL *Nursing theories and models* Springhouse: Springhouse (1992)

Winstead-Fry (ed) *Case studies in nursing theory* New York: National League for Nursing (1986)

Witneben K *Pflegelehrhraft uber Voranssetuingen und perspectiver einerwitisch-honstruhtiven vidalitik der kranhenpfelge* Frankfurt: Verlag Peter Land (1986)

Wolterstorff N *Reason within the bounds of religion* Grand Rapids: Eerdmans (1984)